*The Skidmore-Roth
Outline Series:*

PEDIATRIC NURSING

Leslie Keller, R.N., M.S.N.
Anne Weir, R.N. M.S.N.

Skidmore-Roth Publishing, Inc.

PUBLISHING

Series Editor: Brenda Goodner
Cover design: Veronica Burnett

Notice: The author and the publisher of this volume have taken care
to make certain that all information is correct and compatible with the
standards generally accepted at the time of publication.

Keller, Leslie
Weir, Anne
The Skidmore-Roth Outline Series: Pediatric Nursing/ Leslie Keller,
Anne Weir

ISBN 0-944132-89-8
1. Nursing-Handbooks, Manuals
2. Medical-Handbooks, Manuals

SKIDMORE-ROTH PUBLISHING, INC.
7730 Trade Center Ave.
El Paso, Texas 79912
1(800)825-3150

Table of Contents

9

10

11

12

13

14

Preface

Pediatric patients are a special challenge. They are different psychologically and physiologically and require very special nursing care. Children are also in the process of "becoming" physically, emotionally, and socially. This rapid change affects them not only in terms of physical appearance and function, but also affects the family unit. The pediatric patient is impacted by what occurs in the world around them, family beliefs about child rearing, socioeconomic status, and disease. Any stressor can alter this process of "becoming" and change the outcome -- either positively or negatively -- for that child. In order to provide care for children and their families, the nurse must have an understanding of not only the physiology, pathophysiology, and treatment, but also the impact of illness and stress on the child and the family.

This book is designed as an outline for pediatric patient care. It covers many aspects of that care including growth and development, physical assessment, physiology and pathophysiology as well as treatments and commonly-used medications. It notes the differences between pediatric and adult patients and also addresses psychosocial care and patient/family education. This outline is targeted toward nursing students and nurses who do not practice acute care pediatrics on a regular basis. It is an overall picture of commonly encountered problems and solutions in pediatric nursing.

We would like to thank Patricia Ackerman, R.N., C.P.N.P., Ph.D., Division of Nursing, California State University, Sacramento, California, for her work on the book, especially in the initial stages of manuscript preparation.

We have attempted to provide a reality-based pediatric outline that will provide information based on a "need-to-know" basis. It is designed to heighten awareness of the special challenge that children present. It is our hope that this book will enhance the knowledge base necessary for meeting this challenge.

Leslie S. Keller, R.N., M.S.N.   Anne M. Weir, R.N.P., M.S.N.

1

GROWTH AND DEVELOPMENT

Children were viewed as little more than "small adults" until the late 1800s. They had little relative value in society and were viewed as property. The head of the household had the power of life and death over the children and could determine their fates even into adulthood. Children were expected to behave as adults, and play was viewed as foolish or sinful. Children were workers and began helping out at home at a very early age. Formal schooling was viewed as a luxury and reserved for males only.

Beginning in the late 19th century and continuing today, several theories have attempted to explain the developmental process. Each theorist has studied different aspects of development. Some focused on physical growth and neurological development while others looked at cognitive and "psychosexual" development. Most modern-day practitioners, however, prefer to utilize a combination of the major theories. Information and the central ideas of each of these theorists are presented in the following table.

DEVELOPMENTAL THEORIST AND CENTRAL IDEA			
AGE	*Freud*	*Erikson*	Piaget	*Kohlberg*
Birth - 18 mos.	Oral	Basic Trust vs. Mistrust	Sensorimotor	"Amoral"
18 mos.- 3 years	Anal	Autonomy vs. Shame and Doubt	Symbolic (Preoperational)	Stages 1 - 2
3 - 6 years	Oedipal	Initiative vs. Guilt	Intuition (Preoperational)	Stages 1 - 3
6 - 11 years	Latency	Industry vs. Inferiority	Concrete Operational	Stages 2 - 5
12 - 17 years	Adolescence (genital)	Identity vs. Role Confusion	Formal Operational	Stages 4 - 6
17 - 30 years	Young Adulthood	Intimacy vs. Isolation	Formal Operational	Stages 4 - 6
30 - 60 years	Adulthood	Generativity vs. Stagnation	Formal Operational	Stages 4 - 6
60 years & over	Old Age	Ego Integration vs. Despair	Formal Operational	Stages 4 - 6

Growth and development occurs in regular, related patterns that reflect physical development and the maturation of neuromuscular function. These are termed cephalocaudal, proximodistal, and differentiation. **Cephalocaudal patterns** are exhibited by development that begins on the head. It develops first and is very large and complex while the lower end is simpler and develops later (fetal brain develops first; the head is relatively large compared to the overall size of the infant; there is eye use before hand use; and control over hands is gained before control over feet). **Proximodistal development** is illustrated by the "near-to-far" or "midline to peripheral" concept (limb buds develop before toes and fingers, shoulder control occurs before hand and whole hand is mastered before finger control). CNS development occurs prior to peripheral nervous system development. **Differentiation** is demonstrated by the fact that simple operations/actions develop first and are followed by more complex operations/actions and broad, global behaviors are followed by the more specific and refined patterns (the embryonic development progresses from undifferentiated cell function to highly differentiated, specialized cell function; gross motor function precedes fine motor function).

There is also a definite, predictable sequence in all dimensions of the growth and development process. This allows for the creation of charts with ranges for developmental milestones and growth. **Orderly and continuous sequential patterns** are noted for all children. Each stage of development is affected by the stages preceding it and will influence all future stages (a child learning to walk creeps, crawls, stands, stands alone, and then walks). The theory of **epigenesis** (development results from the growth and differentiation of specialized cells) is also important to the developmental process. New parts and behaviors arise from those already in existence (the nervous system develops from the neural plate, fingers develop from limb buds, and personality facets build on the development of basic trust).

Finally, it must be remembered that growth and development do not occur at the same rate for all children. "There are periods of accelerated growth and periods of decelerated growth in both total body growth and growth of subsystems" (Whaley and Wong, 1988, p. 101). The focus of growth and development changes with different periods during the development of the child. Body proportions change as the child grows.

Each developmental stage is characterized by certain distinct behaviors. These are illustrated in the following table.

STAGE	CHARACTERISTIC BEHAVIORS
Infancy	* Period between birth and 18 months * Rapid physical and social growth * Exhibit generalized, reflexive responses to stimuli * Little meaningful purposeful direction to behavior due to immature cerebral cortex * Born with a series of reflex actions that are predictive of later neurological functioning * Increasing brain size allows for performance of increasingly complex behaviors * Play serves as a practice time for development. Becomes increasingly complex as the infant grows * Cognitive development/functioning is difficult to measure and it is accepted that infants function by operant conditioning
Early Childhood	* Period from 18 months - 4 years * Physical growth has slowed but the systems are maturing and becoming more efficient * Eating habits reflect independence. Food "jags" very common - may become a control issue * Toilet training occurs during this time and often becomes source of anxiety for many parents * Can walk, run, jump and move up and down stairs * Fine motor skills increase * Imitates behavior well as learning continues * Imagination is very active and magical thinking is common * By age 3, vocabulary contains approximately 1000 words * Independence asserted - "terrible twos" seen during this time; the favorite word is "no"

Middle Childhood	* Kindergarten through 3rd grade * Great social and cognitive change * Learning occurring at a rapid rate * As many changes physiologically as an infant * Cerebral dominance and "handedness" established by 4.5 years * Gross motor ability more refined and evidenced by ability to throw a ball with one hand, ride a bicycle, and roller skate * Eye-hand coordination and fine motor skills increase * Play is cooperative and associative. Increased ability to share and cooperate with peers. Games more complex - leader and follower skills develop. Symbolic play important * Cognitive development occurs rapidly. Learn by observation and imitation. Logical thinking and memory increase. Language skills increase * Decrease in egocentric thinking and child more sensitive to others * Self-concept tied to success * Fear bodily harm and injury * Child discovers parents are fallible
Late Childhood	* 8 - 12 years * Continue to mature biologically and physiologically * Girls have growth spurt at about 10 years and are taller and heavier than boys until early adolescence * Gross motor skills more organized and purposeful * Play remains important. Very competitive * Long term memory utilized more as child develops a learning style. Use storytelling to relate events * Sense of humor develops * Independence continues to increase * Heavily rely on parents for praise and support

Adolescence	* Longest period of development
	* Period of great change and turmoil
	* Both sexes experience a growth spurt. May occur any time between 10 and 18 years
	* Epiphyseal plates of long bones close. Governed by sex hormones. Early or late onset of puberty associated with height or mean
	* Body proportions more like those of an adult
	* Apocrine sweat glands and sebaceous glands become active during this time
	* Three types of play:
	  a. Cooperative play (games, clubs, and dating)
	  b. Team play (team sports)
	  c. Construction play (hobbies)
	* Cognitive development continues. Can engage in abstract thinking
	* Search for self-concept continues. Asks what he/she wants to be

Many factors can adversely affect growth and development. The first of these are **genetic factors**. In order to more fully understand how genetic factors interface with growth and development, one must have a basic understanding of embryology. Although the first studies on embryology were done during the golden age of Greece, many "discoveries" have been recent. As embryos develop, 3 distinct phases are apparent. These are cellular multiplication, cellular differentiation, and organ system development. It is also important to remember that all systems arise from 3 primary germ layers. Each system has a critical period during which **any** disruption can adversely affect growth and development. Most system development occurs during the first trimester and coexisting congenital defects most often arise from the same layer. It is not uncommon to see a "grouping" of defects all arising from the same primary germ layer.

GERM LAYER	STRUCTURES ARISING FROM EACH
Mesoderm	* Supporting structure - connective tissue, bones, cartilage, muscle, tendons * Upper portion of urinary system - kidneys and ureters * Reproductive system * Heart and circulatory system * Blood cells
Endoderm	* Linings of GI and respiratory tracts * Tonsils * Parathyroid, thyroid, and thymus glands * Lower urinary tract (bladder and urethra)
Ectoderm	* Nervous system * Skin, hair and nails * Sense organs * Mucous membranes of anus and mouth

Normally, chromosomes exist in pairs (22 pairs of autosomes plus a pair of sex chromosomes). Chromosomal abnormalities include numerical chromosomal abnormalities (monosomy and trisomy) and structural chromosomal abnormalities (translocation and deletion).

Teratogens can have a great impact on developing embryos. A teratogen is defined as any chemical or physical factor that has an adverse effect on a developing embryo or fetus. Exposure to teratogens is inevitable but the amount of damage done, if any, is influenced by the strength of the teratogen, the time during which it is introduced, and its affinity for tissues or specific systems. Many teratogens have predictable consequences. This knowledge of potential fetal damage allows for maternal education on avoidance and prediction of damage should exposure occur.

Physical factors are important to later development. These include genetic mutations (such as cystic fibrosis and sickle cell anemia), diseases that are the result of interaction between genes and the environment (diabetes), and chronic illness or self-care deficits.

Environmental factors such as poor nutrition and environmental hazards and toxins can adversely affect a developing fetus or a growing child. Poor maternal dietary intake often results in intrauterine growth retardation (IUGR) or a small for gestational age (SGA) infant. Many children in the U.S. receive far less than adequate intake of nutrients necessary for physical growth (including brain growth). This adversely affects long-term mental functioning. Environmental hazards such as pollution have been implicated in the development of chronic illness.

Finally, social, cultural, and affective factors must be considered. These include socioeconomic factors, culture, ethnic origin, and religion/religious practices. Health promotion and preventive care are often neglected in lower socioeconomic families. It is difficult to budget for healthcare if it will deprive the family of food or shelter. Insurance is often to expensive for these families. Cultural beliefs about child rearing, health/health promotion, illness, and medical care must be considered when providing care for pediatric patients. These factors determine the type of affection displayed, the expectations of each age and sex, and the way the child is corrected or disciplined. Finally, religion plays an important role in decisions families make when seeking medical care. Some religions have strict guidelines regarding medical care. These include the refusal of blood products and organ transplants by Jehovah's Witnesses and the search for spiritual healing by Christian Scientists.

2

ILLNESS AND HOSPITALIZATION
OF THE PEDIATRIC PATIENT

I.   General Concepts

- Children and their families are affected by illness and hospitalization.

- The pediatric population is at high risk for a variety of illnesses and possible hospitalization due to the immaturity of the body systems and frequent new contacts with other children, animals, and the environment.

- Illness is defined by each individual differently but can be placed on a continuum from wellness to illness.

- Each age group adapts differently to the stressor of illness and/or hospitalization.

- Growth and development levels are important to consider when interacting with the ill child.

- Communication concerning health and illness should be directed toward the parent and child (preschooler and older).

- The family and nurse will play a significant role in maintaining the child's health and optimal functioning level.

- Discharge planning is essential for the pediatric population, since they are dependent on their parents for continued care.

II. Illness

- Can be either acute or chronic

- May require home, outpatient or inpatient care

- May be viewed by toddlers and preschoolers as a punishment for bad behavior

- May hinder normal growth and development if it removes the child from his normal active environment

- Causes stress for family and child

- May be influenced by family views, cultures, ethnicity, social class, financial ability, home environment, community, nutrition

- May occur in any body system

- Nursing Interventions

1. Provide anticipatory guidance to all parents to allow for a sense of control when problems arise.
2. Focus on prevention, detection, education and evaluations, as well as enhancing the child's growth and development during illness.
3. Strive to maintain the child in a normal home environment when disease occurs and attempt to prevent disease progression requiring hospitalization.

III. Hospitalization

Communication

1. Assess Age and Understanding Level of Child
2. Age-Specific Suggestions

a. **Infants** - Use nonverbal communication, discuss with parents procedures, illness. Infants are very aware when parents become upset or fearful and will respond accordingly.

b. **Toddlers and preschoolers** - Very egocentric, need to know what they can do or what will happen to them, let them play with equipment. Give them as much control as possible. They communicate by pulling objects toward them or pushing them away.   Use simple and short sentences, describe things completely and realize they understand everything literally, several explanations may be required.

c. **Schoolage** - Require explanations for everything, communication well-developed but continue to use simple terms, pictures, doll play. Explain what will happen to them, how they can help, and what will happen afterwards.

d. **Adolescents** - Understand all communication but not necessarily medical terms. Utilize pictures, equipment prior to treatments and procedures, encourage questions.

Admission

1. Familiarize child and parent with room, roommate, nurses, and where supplies are stored (diapers, towels, sheets, blankets).
2. Describe hospital routines (change of shifts, times of rounds, mealtimes).
3. Encourage parent and child to do as much for selves and child as is permitted. Give the child as much control over care as possible.
4. Describe all equipment and limitations it poses on child.
5. Inform of safety precautions while in hospital (keeping siderails up, not playing with equipment).
6. Encourage preadmission tours, if possible, to allow for exploring by parent and child in a non-threatening manner.
7. Attempt to staff same nurses to care for child and provide continuity in care.

Medication Administration

1. Explain procedures to parents and child; encouraging questions.
2. Pediatric medication doses are ordered as milligrams/kilogram of body weight. All doses should be checked for accuracy prior to administration. This includes comparison of ordered mg/kg to recommended dose.
3. If only adult doses are available, pediatric doses may be calculated by using Clark's Rule:
   Estimated child's dose = weight of child (lbs) x adult dose

                             150 lbs
4. PO medication:
   a. Position child according to age.
   b. Administer liquids with oral syringe into side of mouth or cheek, or with nipple for infants; and , by spoon or medicine cup for toddlers and older children.
   c. Because it is difficult for young children to swallow pills, medications should be administered in liquid form (elixir or suspension). These may also be used with older children who are unable to swallow pills or capsules.
   d. If administering with food, consider these guidelines:
      - Will the medication alter the taste of the food?
      - Always use a "nonessential" food such as applesauce
      - Mix with only a small amount of food or formula (in case the child takes only a small amount) and feed to the child prior to offering other foods
      - Don't give honey to children under 2 years old to avoid the chance of infantile botulism

IM Injections

1. Assess age and size of child, visualize muscle group to be used.
2. Employ assistance to restrain child as needed to prevent unnecessary trauma.
3. Consider the following muscle groups:
   a. Infants and toddlers: vastus lateralis
   b. Preschoolers: vastus lateralis or dorso gluteal
   c. School-age and adolescents: dorso gluteal, deltoid, ventroguteal
4. Choose the needle length and gauge according to the kind of medication, the amount of medication, and the muscle being injected. The amount of subcutaneous fat, and the viscosity of the medication must be considered.
5. Explain what child should expect and how long it will take.
6. Complete as quickly as possible.
7. Apply a bandaid.
8. Praise the child's attempt to cooperate.

IV Initiation and Maintenance

1. Select site which will be least limiting to patient for age, and which is easily visible for inspection. Sites frequently used include:
   a. Infants: scalp, feet, hands
   b. Toddlers: scalp, non-dominant hand/arm
   c. Preschoolers and older: non-dominant hand or forearm
2. Use non-dominant extremity and allow child to choose site when possible.
3. Explain procedure to child and parent, naming the site, sensations, length of time IV will be in place, and activities child will still be able to do (ambulate, play, shower).
4. Select catheter according to child's size and the viscosity of IV fluid (usually 21-24 gauge is preferred).
5. Prepare all supplies and obtain assistance from other staff with young children who may not be able to cooperate. Allow parents to leave the room if unable to cope with procedure.
6. Secure catheter and tubing (utilize armboards, splints, tape, mitts prn)
7. Monitor site for redness, swelling, induration, or disconnection every 2 hours, provide site care as required by the policy and procedures of the institution.
8. Remember pediatric patients become dehydrated or overhydrated rather quickly, therefore, monitor intake and output, skin status, and lung sounds carefully.
9. Utilize IV pump and Buretrol to allow for closer monitoring of fluid administration and prevention of over or underhydration.

10. Ensure that IV is running according to physician order and within prescribed maintenance rate guidelines:
    - 0 - 10 kg: 100 cc/kg/day
    - >10 - 20 kg: 1000 cc/day for the first 10 kg of body weight plus an additional 50 cc/kg/day for every kg between 10 and 20
    - >20 kg: 1500 cc/day for the first 20 kg of body weight plus an additional 20 cc/kg/day for each kg. greater than 20.
      ** The hourly rate is obtained by dividing the daily volume by 24 hours.
11. If administering IV medications, alter the IV rate to give the medication only as a last resort (volume or time should be changed first)

IV. Treatments and Procedures

1. Explain all treatments and procedures to parents and child.
2. Allow play and experimentation with equipment when possible.
3. Never ask parents to secure child during painful procedure.
4. Special procedures:
   a. LAB WORK
      - Have all materials assembled
      - Explain purpose and procedure to parent and child
      - Secure child and perform procedure as quickly as possible
      - Apply bandaid and pressure
      - Praise child's attempts to cooperate
   b. CATHERIZATION (URINARY)
      - Often very threatening to parent and child
      - Have all materials assembled
      - Explain procedure to parent and child
      - Provide for privacy
      - Secure child and perform procedure as quickly as possible
      - Secure catheter to child and check placement regularly
      - Perform catheter care as required by the policies and procedures of the institution
      - Praise child's attempts to cooperate

V. Stressors From Hospitalization

1. **Reactions According To Age**
   a. **Infants** - Infants adapt well if fed, touched, and cared for; in later infancy they experience separation anxiety, exhibit total body rigidity, protest, detach from parents, exhibit withdrawal behavior.
      - **Nursing Interventions**
        Encourage parents to stay with, visit, and continue routines of home care for infant as much as possible, establish a sense of trust, maintain same nurse assignments, speak to, look at, and

touch infant, provide comfort source as needed (pacifier, bottle, blanket), make environment safe (siderails up, equipment out of reach) attempt to maintain routines, monitor growth and development and provide appropriate interactions and toys.

b. Toddlers - Experience separation anxiety, physically protest and cry, feel a loss of control and rituals, exhibit temper tantrums, exhibit regression, may verbally protest, fear injury and pain, may bite and kick during interaction

   – **Nursing Interventions**:
   Encourage parents to stay with, visit, and continue routines of home care as much as possible, establish trust with parents and child, provide familiar routines and items (security objects), maintain same nurse assignment, allow child a sense of independence, allow child to play and interact with family members, stay with child when parents leave so sense of abandonment is not felt, monitor growth and development and provide appropriate interactions and toys (motor development is important during this age).

c. Preschoolers - Experience separation from family but not to the point of anxiety, fear loss of routines and schedules, sense loss of control, fear bodily injury (very active imagination: fantasy, fears and magical thinking), believe all insides can come out any hole in skin (Bandaid age), exhibit crying, shame, feeling punished, may exhibit regression, aggression, and have nightmares, believe hospitalization is punishment for bad thoughts and actions

   – **Nursing Interventions**:
   Encourage parents to stay or visit frequently, encourage parents to call child on the phone, provide familiar routines and allow independence in daily care as much as possible, maintain same nurse assignment, allow child to interact and play with others and family, keep night light on during sleep, allow familiar items to be kept with child, explain in simple terms what procedures are going to be done just prior to being done, praise child for accomplishments, utilize play therapy as much as possible to diminish fears, encourage interaction and play with other children in the hospital in age group, monitor growth and development.

d. Schoolage - Experience fear of separation from family and friends, getting behind in school, body mutilation, and loss of independence; exhibit stress by attempting to negotiate, crying, fighting, withdrawal, attempting to be brave, ask many questions

   – **Nursing Interventions**:
   Describe illness, treatments, and procedures to child and parent, encourage family visitation, encourage phone calls, letters, banners from friends and family, allow questions and answer in simple terms, allow independence and choices as much as possible, encourage doing school work, set limits, establish routines, utilize play therapy, tell child crying is O.K., provide child with privacy after procedures to recompose self, encourage rooming

with or playing with other children of the same age, monitor growth and development.

   e. Adolescents - Experience fear of being different, embarrassment, bodily injury, separation from family and friends, loss of privacy, loss of independence, may exhibit overconfidence, withdrawal, noncompliance with regimens, regression, and acting out

       – **Nursing Interventions**
          Maintain honest and open communication, provide information regarding illness and treatments, encourage questions and provide understandable answers, provide privacy, encourage interaction with family, friends and others in age group who are hospitalized, assist with maintaining homework, allow decision making as possible, set limits.

Nursing Care for Pediatric Patients

1. Stressors

   a. Altered body image - Assist with hygiene and care, assess child's self-concept, have child color/draw a picture of self and discuss, ask what would make them feel better and look better and assist with reaching goal.

   b. Fear of death - Assess level of understanding and discuss concerns.

   Infants - No concept of death, may note separation if loved one dies, unaware that own illness could lead to death

       – **Nursing Interventions:** Support parents, provide information, determine what religious ceremonies are appropriate if infant dies. If infant dies, allow parent to hold child in quiet room, provide a photograph of infant, lock of hair and footprints (if parents do not have these). Utilize infant's name when speaking about infant, actively listen to parents.

   Toddlers - No concept of death, may sense separation and impact on routines, may want to visit dead relative, unaware that illness may cause death

       – **Nursing Interventions:** Support parents and child if illness is terminal, provide parents time for questions regarding child's status and give honest answers, provide parents time alone with toddler, utilize toddler's name when speaking of toddler after death, listen.

   Preschoolers - Believe death is temporary and reversible, a time of "sleeping", believe all body functions continue after death, believe illness or death can happen if someone is "bad"; fear how they will go to the bathroom or eat after death; wonder if they will be cold, hungry or be able to play, fear it will hurt to die, may ask if they are going to die due to illness.

   – **Nursing Interventions**: Support parent and child if illness is terminal, identify child's beliefs about death and clarify misconcep-
   tions utilizing words and terms they can understand, provide
   comfort and honesty to child and parents, after death allow parent
   to visit and hold child, ask if there is anything they would like
   done, actively listen to parents.

Schoolage

6 - 9 years - Personify death (bogeyman), think of death concretely
and may wonder if they are going to die when sick, realize body will
decay once dead and that death is permanent

9 - 10 years - Full concept of death develops, may fear own death
and see it as unfair, may become aggressive if own death is near,
may try to appear strong and unafraid in front of parents, may fear
people will see them naked or soil themselves once dead, may ask
about what happens after life

   – **Nursing Interventions:** Encourage parent to openly discuss illness and death with child, ask child what death means to them
   and discuss feelings and fears, encourage parents to allow child
   as much independence as possible before death, incorporate
   child in planning of "will" after death and support parents and
   child's wishes before and after death, allow parent to hold child
   after death or stay in quiet room, actively listen to parents.

Adolescents - Well-developed concept of death, thinks it won't happen to him, may still have some magical thinking (death as punishment), may become angry, frustrated, experience denial or become
withdrawn when confronted with death.

   – **Nursing Interventions:** Support adolescent and parent, give
   honest, and thorough information, allow adolescent to discuss
   feelings and wishes or dreams he would like to achieve before
   death, encourage interaction with other adolescents and friends,
   allow adolescent to make decisions, as possible; encourage
   adolescent to assist making plans for after death (what he will
   wear, flowers), allow parents time with adolescent before and
   after death, actively listen.

Families of a terminally-ill child - Parents need special support,
they often tend to overprotect child and encourage dependency of
child on themselves, may isolate selves from spouse, other children
or society; need time to talk, ask questions, and go through the grieving process, may abandon the dying child.

   – **Nursing Interventions:** Listen to family, encourage parents to assist with daily care of child, encourage parents to treat child as
   "normal", provide family with support group to discuss feelings, assess how each member is coping with stress and discuss heal-
   thier ways to cope as needed, give family as much control of child
   in hospital as possible, let family know you care.

 c. **Interruptions in routines** - Assess patient's daily home routines
    (meals, voiding, play, school, baths), and attempt to incorporate into

hospital care, allow as much independence and decision-making as possible, discuss with child what would make hospitalization better for them.

d. **Interruption in school** - Utilize playroom or schoolroom and teachers as available, allow time for school work, encourage reading, writing, and ask child questions pertaining to school, allow child to interact/play with other children their age, encourage visits, letters from schoolmates and teachers.

e. **Isolation** - Utilize washable toys, books, television, telephone, coloring books in room, explain necessity of isolation and length, encourage visits by parents; talk to, touch and spend time with child, play games or other activities which promote interaction.

f. **Loneliness -** Prevent by introducing child to others in age group, allow child to go to playroom, encourage utilization of telephone, writing letters, provide as much interaction as possible, allow child to discuss feelings and suggest ways that might help them cope with the loneliness.

g. **Pain** - Assess location, frequency, duration, and cause; differentiate between physiological and psychological pain, use pain scales such as Wong-Baker faces, numerical analog, or pain thermometer. Always assess effectiveness of pain medications.

   - **Infants** - Will display change in vital signs, and withdrawal of area in pain; administer medications as ordered, reposition, stroke, swaddle, rock, talk to, infants unable to localize and communicate where discomfort is, determine and record effectiveness of interventions

   - **Toddlers** - Will display change in vital signs, have child point to and describe pain, utilize a face scale to monitor degree of pain and how child feels, document location and degree of pain and alleviating activities, medicate as ordered, hold, reposition, allow play and movement, determine and record effectiveness of interventions

   - **Preschoolers** - Will display change in vital signs, have child identify site and intensity or sensation, what would make them feel better, evaluate using face scale, utilize repositioning, distraction, imagery and pain medications as needed, hold/stroke child, keep environment quiet and non-threatening, allow play and movement, determine and record effectiveness of interventions

   - **Schoolage** - Have child identify site and intensity, assess pain using a rating scale (0-10), or other descriptive pain scale, reposition, utilize imagery, distractions, pain medication as needed, determine and record effectiveness of intervention

   - **Adolescents** - Have patient identify site, intensity, duration and sensation, utilize repositioning, imagery, distraction and pain medication as ordered, determine and record effectiveness of interventions

    h. Restraints - Provide 10 minutes each hour in which movement is allowed, maintain movement in as many extremities as possible, provide age appropriate stimulation:

- **Infants:** Mobiles, busy box, tapes, touching, rocking
- **Toddlers:** Busy boxes, noise makers, allow to walk every hour when awake
- **Preschoolers, schoolage, and adolescents:** Explain need for restraints, length of use, and limitation; provide colors, TV, books, musical instruments, and interaction as diversional activities

    i. Restricted diet/NPO - Continue thorough mouth care, discourage parent from bringing in food or eating in front of child, limit discussion of food, provide other activities during regular mealtime, discuss length and limitations of food/fluid restrictions

VI. Play Therapy

1. Play room should be a safe haven, no procedures should be performed in this area.
2. Play should be a part of every child's daily routines.
3. Play is an excellent outlet for childhood anxiety and energy.
4. Play should be age appropriate and meet safety requirements.

VII. Discharge Planning

1. The nurse should begin preparing the parent and child for discharge, beginning on the day of admission.
2. Discharge planning should be a daily progression so that the family and child are prepared to go home when the physician discharges the child.
3. Items to include in making an assessment for discharge:
   a. Physical needs at home
   b. Ability to perform ADLs
   c. Home environment
   d. Special care needs (medication administration, PT, OT)
   e. Special nutritional requirements
   f. Psychological needs of child and family
   g. Learning needs of child and family
   h. Family's ability to care for child once discharged
4. Items to include in teaching:
   a. Explanation of disorder
   b. Specific care required for disorder
   c. Correct medication administration (drug, dose, route, time and side effects)
   d. Signs and symptoms which require parents to seek medical attention

    e. Phone number to call to seek medical attention

    f. How to get help in case of emergency

    g. Date of next follow-up appointment

3

RESPIRATORY DISORDERS

I. General Concepts

- The respiratory system is composed of the oropharynx, nasopharynx, larynx, trachea, bronchi, bronchioles, lungs and alveoli.

- The pediatric respiratory system continues to mature after birth.

- The infant's respiratory tract is more susceptible to obstruction than the adult's due to these differences in anatomy: greater soft palate, larger tongue, larger amounts of soft tissue in airway. These anatomical differences predispose infants to greater risk of obstruction if airway becomes swollen. Alveoli continue to mature after birth.

- Infants are nose breathers and utilize the diaphragm to breathe; therefore, nasal obstruction can cause anoxia in infancy.

- Signs that indicate respiratory difficulty include: coughing, wheezing, rhinorrhea, irritability or nervousness, tachypnea. As severity progresses respiratory distress may occur and is recognized by anxiety, nasal flaring, use of accessory muscles for respiration, (causing retractions), paleness, cyanosis, grunting, tachycardia, irritability. Prompt treatment is required to prevent respiratory collapse and failure.

- Whether disorders are acute or chronic, they may be life-threatening, and require prompt treatment.

II. Specific Respiratory Disorders

Congenital Defects

1. CYSTIC FIBROSIS (CF)

a. Description - An autosomal recessive disorder in which there is over-production of mucous by the exocrine glands. The excess viscous mucous affects the lungs, small intestines, pancreas and bile ducts. It is a progressive disease process which eventually leads to an early death, usually by late twenties. It is the number one cause of genetically-related death in Caucasian children.

b. Signs and Symptoms - Symptoms may or may not be present initial-ly. Pulmonary signs include coughing, tachypnea, retractions (infan-cy), bronchial plugging, pneumothorax, increased number of respiratory infections, pulmonary function test that indicate increased residual volume, increased total lung capacity, decreased vital capacity and decreased flow rates, dyspnea, wheezing, atelectasis, productive coughing. Gastrointestinal signs include: meconium ileus (newborn), loose stools, poor weight gain, chronic diarrhea, vora-cious appetite, abdominal distension, prolapse of rectum, intestinal obstruction, steatorrhea, azotorrhea, pancreatic insufficiency, gastroesophageal reflux, gallstones.

c. Diagnostic Procedures - Pilocarpine iontophoresis for sweat electrolytes reveals chloride greater than 60mg/L, pancreatic enzyme evaluation shows decreased levels present, fat absorption assess-ment reveals diminished fat absorption present, and family history positive for CF

d. Medical Interventions

– **Medications** - Administration of pancreatic enzymes (Pancrease), bronchodilators, long-term suppressive antibiotic therapy, in-creased salt intake, Pulmozyme

– **Treatments** - Maintain healthy pulmonary functioning (CPT, hydra-tion, pulmonary toilet); provide diet which is 130-150% greater than normal caloric needs with fat content 30% of total calories; adequate salt intake; provide multivitamins, vitamin E, K, D, and calcium

– **Surgery** - Unnecessary

e. Nursing Interventions

– **Assessment and Actions**

• Assess child's respiratory and nutritional status.

• Monitor child's weight every day.

• During hospitalization monitor vital signs, respiratory status, hydration status, comfort level, and prevent further infections.

• Ensure respiratory treatments are done.

- Encourage healthy diet.
- Administer medications as ordered.
- Encourage exercise (swimming, walking, jogging) and alternate with rest periods at home.
- Assess for signs indicating potential complications.
- Refer parents to genetic counseling.
- If patient is an adolescent or young adult, refer for genetic counseling and information regarding contraception.

- **Teaching**
  - Explain diagnosis to parent and child.
  - Explain treatment regimen:
    1. Administer pancreatic enzymes regularly with meals to enhance absorption.
    2. Provide high calorie, high protein foods in diet, as well as vitamin supplements.
    3. Encourage liberal use of salt on foods, especially in hot climates.
    4. Monitor child's weight weekly.
  - Teach parents and child CPT, postural drainage, oxygen therapy and positioning to promote clearing of lung fields; encourage fluid intake prior to treatment to loosen secretions.
  - Instruct child in breathing exercise and assist with selecting regular times to perform.
  - Teach parent and child about medications prescribed (drug, dose, route, time, and side effects) and how to use inhaler.

- **Emotional Care**
  - Promote growth and development and encourage child to do as much for self as possible.
  - Discuss chronicity of disease and how child and family are coping.
  - Provide emotional support to family and child.
  - Provide support group information to family.

f. **Potential Complications** - Malabsorption syndrome, emphysema, rectal prolapse, cirrhosis, portal hypertension, respiratory infections, spontaneous pneumothorax, death

Acquired Defects

1. ASTHMA (BRONCHIAL)

a. **Description** - A reversible, obstructive airway disease associated with airway irritability and bronchospasm, which causes trapping of air in the bronchioles. It may be intermittent or chronic and may be due to an allergic reaction or have a genetic link. It leads to respiratory acidosis if left untreated. It is often the great imitator of other disease processes and, therefore, it is important to rule out foreign-body obstruction, cystic fibrosis, and congestive heart failure before diagnosis is confirmed. It is the most common illness in childhood and is responsible for more missed school days than any other illness.

b. Signs and Symptoms - Acute or gradual onset of expiratory wheezing, chest tightness, retractions, tachypnea, nonproductive coughing with or without wheezing, cyanosis, diaphoresis, nervousness, altered mental status; child may position self over table or chair leaning forward to ease respiratory efforts

c. Diagnostic Procedures - Diagnosed by history, physical findings, presence of elevated pCO_2, CXR usually not helpful unless to rule out obstruction; sweat chloride test utilized to rule out CF, immunological assay tests reveal elevated IgE, pulmonary function test utilized to determine whether hospitalization necessary

d. Medical Interventions
 - **Medications** - Administer oxygen, terbutaline, isoetharine, aminophylline, antihistamines, hydrocortisone, Cromolyn sodium, steroids (prednisone, beclomethasone)
 - **Treatments** - Identify and remove causative agent, improve pulmonary function by medication, teach breathing exercises, increase hydration by IV, maintain normal lifestyle and promote exercise.
 - **Surgery** - Unnecessary

e. Nursing Interventions
 - **Assessment and Actions**
   • Assess and evaluate level of distress and position child for comfort and to facilitate breathing.
   • Monitor vital signs.
   • Assist family in identifying causative agent or cause of exacerbation (allergy testing, stress reduction).
   • Assist child and family in identifying early warning signs of attack (itchy throat, "funny" feeling in chest, nervousness, paleness) and to take immediate action, including medication administration, positioning child to enhance breathing, promote rest and fluids.
   • Monitor child for therapeutic response and/or untoward effects of medication.
   • Assess for signs indicating potential complications (sudden decrease in wheezing, drop in PaO_2 or increase in $PaCO_2$, downward trend in oxygen saturations).
 - **Teaching**
   • Explain diagnosis to parent and child.
   • Prepare child and family for treatment regimen (medication administration, oxygen therapy, rehydration) and instruct on importance of each.

- Teach parents and child correct use of metered dose inhaler and obtain return demonstration; discuss when to use inhaler and action to take if relief not obtained after use.
- Teach child breathing exercises to extend expiratory time and increase expiratory effort.
- Teach parent about medication prescribed (drug, dose, route, time, and side effects). Instruct that the medication regimen is very strict and medications must be given exactly as prescribed.
- Emphasize to parents the importance of prompt treatment when an attack occurs.

  – **Emotional Care**
  - Promote normal growth and development.
  - Provide support to family and child.
  - Provide support group information to family.

  f. **Potential Complications** - Infection, collapsed lung, emphysema, atelectasis; status asthmaticus (the body's inability to respond to the treatment regimen for asthma.) This condition requires emergency treatment. Signs of respiratory distress increase and metabolic acidosis occurs; treatment focuses on administration of IV epinephrine, aminophylline, isoproterenol, oxygen therapy, IV fluids, resuscitation, treatment of acidosis, monitoring vital signs and providing support to family and child. This can be fatal if not treated.

2. **BRONCHIOLITIS**

   a. **Description** - An inflammation of the bronchioles accompanied by mucous obstruction. It is usually caused by the respiratory synctial virus and affects children less than two years of age. It can be fatal if left untreated.

   b. **Signs and Symptoms** - Usually acute in onset; history of upper respiratory infection for several days, rhinorrhea, shallow respirations; dry, harsh, cough; retractions, cyanosis, fever, crackles, grunting, nasal flaring, expiratory wheezes, loss of appetite, tachypnea, diminished breath sounds and atelectasis on auscultation; may be associated with otitis media and/or pneumonia

   c. **Diagnostic Procedures** - Diagnosis is determined by physical findings, presence of hyperinflation of lungs, retractions, ruling out asthma, as well as obtaining a positive culture for the respiratory syncitial virus (RSV).

   d. **Medical Interventions**
   - **Medications** - Administer bronchodilators (may not be effective in infants), epinephrine, oral steroids, Ribavirin (only if RSV infection confirmed)
   - **Treatments** - Maintain airway, prevent secondary infection, administer oxygen, fluids, and perform intubation if severe

symptoms present; hospitalization may be required if dehydration, secondary bacterial infection or respiratory distress occur.

- **Surgery** - Unnecessary

e. Nursing Interventions

- **Assessment and Actions**
  - Assess child's vital signs, hydration status, and be alert for increasing signs of respiratory distress.
  - Administer medications, oxygen (via nasal cannula, oxygen hood or ET tube), and fluids.
  - Maintain quiet environment.
  - Keep child in contact isolation and utilize thorough handwashing.
  - Assess for signs indicating potential complications.

- **Teaching**
  - Explain diagnosis and treatment regimen to parents.
  - Teach parents about medication prescribed (drug, dose, route, time and side effects).
  - Teach parents about isolation. Emphasize necessity in following isolation regimen. Instruct that this limits spread of RSV to others as it is not as fragile as other viruses and may live up to 48 hours on inanimate objects such as clothing.

- **Emotional Care**
  - Promote growth and development while hospitalized.
  - Provide support to parents and child.

f. Potential Complications - Secondary respiratory infection, hypoxia, death (in severe untreated cases)

3. BRONCHOPULMONARY DYSPLASIA (BPD)

a. **Description** - A chronic lung disorder in which there is hypertrophy of small airways, squamous metaplasia and fibrosis of the alveoli and bronchioles. The alveoli collapse and air movement is trapped. It occurs in infants who require prolonged mechanical ventilation with high oxygen tensions (increased PIP).

b. **Signs and Symptoms** - Signs of respiratory distress, tachypnea, tachycardia, cyanosis on room air, long-term oxygen dependency, growth and developmental delays, difficulty feeding, barrel-chest appearance (in long-term disorder), inability to wean from mechanical ventilation

c. **Diagnostic Procedures** - Diagnosed by birth history, X-ray reveals hyperaeration and atelectasis, ABG reveals hypoxia or compensating hypercarbia, acidosis, and mild hypoxemia; echocardiogram shows right ventricular hypertrophy

d. Medical Interventions

- **Medications** - Administer oxygen, theophylline, terbutaline, isoproterenol, diuretics, steroids, surfactant replacement therapy (at delivery in preterm infants)
- **Treatments** - Monitor oxygenation using transcutaneous PaO_2, provide positive pressure ventilation, increase nutritional intake, and maintain hydration status
- **Surgery** - Unnecessary

e. Nursing Interventions

- **Assessment and Actions**
  - Assess child's vital signs, respiratory, hydration, electrolyte and nutritional status; assess carefully for signs and symptoms of viral respiratory infections (chronically-ill infants have increased susceptibility).
  - Be prepared for intubation.
  - Prepare parents for long-term therapy (usually resolves by 3-4 years).
  - Assess signs indicating potential complications.

- **Teaching**
  - Explain diagnosis and treatment regimen to family.
  - Prepare for home care by teaching signs of respiratory distress to parents and teaching them when to seek medical help.
  - Teach parents about medications prescribed (drug, dose, route, time and side effects).
  - Teach signs and symptoms of infection and to avoid contact with persons with known infections.

- **Emotional Care**
  - Promote growth and development and promote rest.
  - Provide support to family and child.

f. Potential Complications - Infection, congestive heart failure, respiratory failure, pneumothorax, chronic respiratory disease (lifelong), long-term developmental and growth retardation, death

4. EPIGLOTTITIS (ACUTE)

a. Description - A bacterial infection of the epiglottis causing edema and inflammation. It is a rapidly progressing disorder and is a medical emergency. It must be treated promptly before complete airway obstruction occurs. This disorder is typically seen among children 3-6 years old. It is most commonly caused by *H. influenza* Type B.

b. Signs and Symptoms - Initial onset may be quite subtle with increasing restlessness. As the condition progresses signs and symptoms include: inspiratory stridor, high fever, muffled voice, barking cough, sore throat. If untreated, inspiratory stridor, tachypnea, fear, retractions, dysphagia, excessive drooling, respiratory distress and obstruction occur. Typically child assumes a "tripod" position supporting

body with hands with chin thrust forward and mouth open in attempt to open airway wider.

c. **Diagnostic Procedures** - Diagnosed by physical assessment, lateral x-ray reveals enlarged or thumb-like epiglottis. Quick ventilation may be required via intubation, then the swollen, cherry red epiglottis can be seen.

d. **Medical Interventions**
   – **Medications** - Administer antibiotics (ampicillin, chloramphenicol).
   – **Treatments** - Maintain open airway by artificial airway placement and provide fluid resuscitation as needed. Prepare to intubate.
   – **Surgery** - Tracheostomy may be necessary, especially if intubation is not possible.

e. **Nursing Interventions**
   – **Assessment and Actions**
      • Be alert to signs and symptoms and treat promptly.
      • Assist with intubation or tracheostomy and secure tube.
      • Assess vital signs, hydration status, ABGs, comfort level.
      • Administer antibiotics as ordered.
      • Determine method in which child can communicate.
      • Once extubated, monitor respiratory status and offer fluids.
      • Assess for signs indicating potential complications.
   – **Teaching**
      • Explain diagnosis and need for emergency treatment.
      • Teach parents about medications prescribed (drug, dose, route, time, and side effects).
   – **Emotional Care**
      • Encourage parents to remain with child until child is calm.
      • Provide support to family and child and reassure that treatment is focused on reducing the size of the epiglottis and maintaining airway function.

f. **Potential Complications** - Death from occlusion of airway

5. **FOREIGN BODY ASPIRATION (FBA)**
   a. **Description** - A partial or complete blockage of the airway. It is typically seen in infants and toddlers. It may be life-threatening and is often due to ingestion of small items (raisins, peanuts, gum, popcorn).
   b. **Signs and Symptoms** - Depends on whether partial or complete obstruction has occurred and on location; partial obstruction symptoms include choking, coughing, wheezing, gagging, whistling sound on inspiration, diminished breath sounds or chest movement on affected side, cyanosis; complete obstruction of upper airway causes absence of breathing, nervousness, fainting, severe cyanosis and eventual death, if left untreated.

    c. Diagnostic Procedures - Diagnosed by history, physical examination, x-ray reveals lodged item or trapped air, bronchoscopy may be used to visualize, confirm, or retrieve item.

    d. Medical Interventions

        – **Medications** - Administer oxygen and antibiotics after removal.

        – **Treatments** - Partial obstruction requires removal by bronchoscopy or laryngoscopy; complete obstruction requires the Heimlich Maneuver or emergency intubation.

        – **Surgery** - Tracheostomy placement may be necessary to open airway.

    e. Nursing Interventions

        – **Assessment and Actions**

          • Assist with prompt diagnosis and administer emergency treatment.

          • Prepare child for sedation and anesthesia if bronchoscopy or laryngoscopy required.

          • Describe necessity of tracheostomy to parents and what to expect if tracheostomy placement required.

          • Assess vital signs, respiratory status, keep environment calm, keep patient NPO initially after removal of object.

          • Avoid treatments or activities which may cause further irritation to respiratory system (CPT, coughing).

          • Assess for signs indicating potential complications.

        – **Teaching**

          • Explain diagnosis to parents and discuss treatment required.

          • Discuss safety in home and identify appropriate items to allow child to have in hand.

          • Teach parents CPR before discharged.

          • Teach parents about medication prescribed (drug, dose, route, time, and side effects).

        – **Emotional Care**

          • Provide support to family and child.

          • Provide time for grieving and refer to counseling if death occurs.

    f. Potential Complications - Swelling of airway after removal, erosion of airway if undetected initially, infection, if hypoxic for several minutes may cause brain damage and/or death.

6. LARYNGOTRACHEOBRONCHITIS (LTB)

    a. Description - A viral respiratory infection that has a sudden onset. It causes inflammation and swelling of the laryngeal area and usually occurs in the toddler age group. It is the most common form of croup and is more common in boys than girls. It is most commonly caused by parainfluenza 1,2, and 3 viruses, respiratory syncytial virus, and rhinovirus.

b. **Signs and Symptoms** - Symptoms occur more commonly at night and during cold seasons. History of upper respiratory infection, hoarseness, barking cough, retractions, inspiratory stridor, diminished breath sounds, mild fever, crackles, rhonchi, cyanosis, tachycardia, nervousness; differentiated from acute spasmodic croup by slower, more gradual onset

c. **Diagnostic Procedures** - Diagnosed by reviewing history, ruling out epiglottitis by lateral neck x-ray; visual inspection reveals subglottal narrowing

d. **Medical Interventions**
   – **Medications** - May administer corticosteroids (not generally indicated and controversial), nebulized racemic epinephrine if hospitalized, Ribavarin (only if RSV infection confirmed), antibiotics if secondary bacterial infection (i.e. otitis media) present
   – **Treatments** - Maintain airway, provide humidified oxygen administration, monitor for continued airway difficulty and distress, rehydrate, may require intubation if symptoms not relieved.
   – **Surgery** - Unnecessary

e. **Nursing Interventions**
   – **Assessment and Actions**
     • Assist with prompt diagnosis.
     • If hospitalized, assess vital signs, respiratory efforts and for progressive worsening; monitor I & O, have intubation equipment at hand, administer oxygen as ordered and monitor oxygenation.
     • Assess for signs indicating potential complications.
   – **Teaching**
     • Explain diagnosis to parents and discuss treatment regimen.
     • If child treated at home, discuss with parents signs of increasing respiratory difficulty and when to seek further medical assistance; encourage using humidifier and keeping child quiet in bed.
     • Instruct parents to offer fluids liberally unless potential for aspiration.
     • Prepare parents for coughing or vomiting of mucous after crises resolved.
     • Teach parents about medication prescribed (drug, dose, route, time, and side effects).
   – **Emotional Care**
     • Provide quiet activities in bed appropriate for age.
     • Encourage parents to stay with child and instruct them to keep child under tent if hospitalized.

- Provide support to family and child.

f. Potential Complications - Recurrence, infection, death if severe and untreated

7. RESPIRATORY DISTRESS SYNDROME (RDS)

a. Description - A progression in alveolar insufficiency and collapse that causes atelectasis, hypoxemia, and respiratory compromise. It is seen in preterm infants and is due to insufficient surfactant production. It was previously know as hyaline membrane disease (HMD).

b. Signs and Symptoms - Initially at birth symptoms absent but infant quickly (30 minutes to 2 hours postdelivery) exhibits respiratory symptoms: retractions, nasal flaring, tachypnea, grunting, cyanosis, apnea while on room air; leads to metabolic and respiratory acidosis.

c. Diagnostic Procedures - Diagnosed by history, ABGs reveals increased CO_2, and x-ray of lung field which shows atelectasis (ground-glass appearance) and air filled bronchioles.

d. Medical Interventions
- **Medications** - Administer oxygen via artificial airway (ET tube, nasal prongs) prn, administer replacement surfactant at delivery before first breath; may administer pharmacological paralyzing agents (pancuronium or vecuronium) and sedative agents (morphine sulfate, ativan, fentanyl, and demerol)
- **Treatments** - Maintain respiratory function, correct acidosis, prevent complications, provide sedation, monitor nutrition and fluid status
- **Surgery** - May be necessary to correct a patent ductus arteriosus (PDA) which has not closed after delivery and causes a left to right shunting of blood from aorta to pulmonary arteries thus prolonging respiratory problems

e. Nursing Interventions
- **Assessment and Actions**
  - Assess preterm infant after birth for respiratory problems and obtain prompt interventions from physician.
  - Monitor administration of oxygen and maintain airway.
  - Assess vital signs, respiratory status.
  - Maintain neutral thermal environment to decrease metabolic requirements.
  - Maintain minimal stimulation policy (quiet environment, low lighting, minimal handling).
  - Monitor for signs and symptoms of PDA ("washing machine" murmur, bounding peripheral pulses, increased oxygen/respiratory support demands, and decreased ability to wean from respiratory support).
  - Assess nutritional needs and monitor growth pattern.

- Provide appropriate developmental intervention as infant's condition allows.
- Encourage parental participation in care and decision making.
- Monitor carefully for signs and symptoms of infection and oxygen toxicity.
- Assess for signs indicating potential complications.
- If mother planning to breastfeed, encourage her to utilize a breast pump until infant's status improves.

  - **Teaching**
    - Discuss diagnosis and treatment regimen with family.
    - Prepare family for what to expect child to look like (monitors, tubing, IV sites, sounds).
  - **Emotional Care**
    - Provide support to family and child.
    - Promote bonding.
    - Allow parents to visit as much as possible.

  f. **Potential Complications** - BPD, infections, retinopathy of prematurity (damage to the retina due to excessive oxygenation), intraventricular hemorrhage, pneumothorax, pulmonary interstitial emphysema (PIE), pneumopericardium, vena cava syndrome (due to increased pressure in thorax that decreases blood return to heart), necrotizing enterocolitis (NEC), death

8. PNEUMONIA

  a. **Description** - A viral or bacterial pulmonary infection occurring frequently in infancy and early childhood. It may be a primary disease or be the result of another illness. It is manifested by inflammation and consolidation of pulmonary parenchyma. It is classified by the causative agent with viral being more common (most often respiratory syncytial virus). The bacterial form is caused most often by pneumococci, streptococci, staphylococci, or chlamydia. Pneumococcal is most often spread by respiratory droplet in winter and early spring; chlamydial is severe, diffuse and often difficult to treat; staphylococcal often is the primary infection (usually nosocomial in origin); and, streptococcal lobular, less common, is spread via the lymphatic system.

  b. **Signs and Symptoms** - Viral: acute or insidious onset, slight or severe cough, slow to high grade fever, malaise to lethargy. Bacterial: abrupt onset, lethargy, preceded by viral infection, respiratory distress, shocky appearance, decreased breath sounds, coarse crackles, friction rub, use of accessory muscles, nasal discharge

  c. **Diagnostic Procedures** - Viral: CXR reveals diffuse infiltrates; Bacterial: CXR shows patchy consolidation of one or more lobes, pneumatoceles (staph) or pleural effusions (strep)

   d. Medical Interventions

- **Medications** - Antibiotics, antipyretics, IV fluid
- **Treatments** - Maintain patent airway, fever reduction, oxygen, pulmonary hygiene (CPT, updrafts)
- **Surgery** - Unnecessary

   e. Nursing Interventions

- **Assessment and Actions**
  - Be alert to signs and symptoms of increasing respiratory distress/failure.
  - Monitor for loss of patent airway.
  - Assess vital signs, hydration status, ABGs, comfort level.
  - Assess effectiveness of antibiotic and antipyretic therapy.
  - Assess effectiveness of oxygen therapy.
  - Assist with diagnostic procedures and maintenance of good pulmonary hygiene.

- **Teaching**
  - Explain meaning of diagnosis and planned medical treatment plan including all medications prescribed.
  - Explain signs, symptoms and prevention of recurrence.
  - Explain when to seek additional medical treatment (if not hospitalized).

- **Emotional Care**
  - Encourage parents to remain with child.
  - Provide support to child and family. Assure parents that onset of pneumonia is often sudden and provide positive reinforcement for seeking care.

   f. Potential Complications - Secondary infection, respiratory failure, dehydration, febrile seizures, atelectasis, pulmonary abscesses, pneumothorax, death.

9. TONSILLITIS (STREPTOCOCCAL PHARYNGITIS)

   a. Description - An inflammation and formation of edema of the lymphoid tissue (tonsils) in the palatine or pharyngeal area of the mouth. It is frequently caused by Group A Beta hemolytic streptococci and is commonly seen in childhood.

   b. Signs and Symptoms - Reddened swollen tonsils (may become so enlarged that they block passageway of air), sore throat, difficulty swallowing, hoarseness or muffling of voice, fever; may be accompanied by otitis media, sinusitis, skin rash or peritonsillar abscesses. May progress to meningitis, rheumatic fever, or acute glomerulonephritis.

   c. Diagnostic Procedures - Diagnosed by inspection and obtaining positive throat culture, ASO titer also increased.

d. Medical Interventions

- **Medications** - Administration of antibiotic (penicillin G, erythromycin or clindamycin) and antipyretics
- **Treatments** - Promote gargling with warm salt water if mild, bedrest, increased fluid intake; if surgery required prevent sucking activity postoperatively.
- **Surgery** - Surgical removal of tonsils if blocking airway or if recurrent inflammation occurs (tonsillectomy).

e. Nursing Interventions

- **Assessment and Actions**
  - Assist with obtaining throat culture.
  - Assess vital signs, hydration status, and comfort level.
  - Position patient prone or on side postoperatively to prevent pooling of blood in back of throat.
  - Assess for signs of hemorrhage postoperatively (frequent swallowing, vomiting frank blood, pallor).
  - Prevent irritation to surgical area (prevent coughing, avoid use of straw, serve only bland foods when off NPO status).
  - Promote oral hydration postoperatively by offering cool drinks, jello, ice chips, nonacidic drinks.
  - Encourage high fluid intake to prevent crusting of incision - if wound crusts over and breaks off, hemorrhage can occur.
  - Provide method for reducing discomfort.
  - Assess for signs indicating potential complications.

- **Teaching**
  - Discuss diagnosis and treatment regimen with parents and child.
  - If home care prescribed, discuss with parents antibiotic administration, antipyretic administration, increasing fluid intake, gargling with warm salt water, utilizing vaporizor.
  - If tonsillectomy required, prepare child and family for procedure and postoperative care.
  - Prepare family and child for discharge after surgery (omit sucking, spicy or hot foods or fluids) and teach them signs that would indicate bleeding.

- **Emotional Care**
  - Provide support to family.

f. Potential Complications - Postoperative hemorrhaging, occlusion of airway if severe edema develops

4

CARDIOVASCULAR DISORDERS

I. General Concepts

- The heart is completely formed by the eighth week of fetal development.

- The heart is composed of four chambers, 2 atria and 2 ventricles.

- At birth, once the umbilical cord is clamped off, the pressure changes within the circulatory system causing the heart to begin functioning independently of maternal circulation.

- The infant's heart is larger in proportion to the body than that of the adult's.

- The heart grows throughout childhood and reaches adult size by the end of adolescence.

- Pressure in the normal heart is greater on the left side than on the right.

- Heart defects may be either congenital or acquired.

II. Specific Cardiovascular Disorders

Congenital Heart Defects

- Cardiac defects that exist from birth

- May be undetected or life-threatening depending upon the nature of the defect

- May be caused by maternal illness, maternal drug ingestation, maternal age (over 40), hereditary factors, or unknown etiology

- May be accompanied by other defects

- May cause: increased cardiac workload, pulmonary hypertension, diminished cardiac output, hypoxemia, cardiomegaly, altered growth and development, decreased activity tolerance, tachypnea, clubbing of fingers and toes, poor weight gain, poor feeding

- May be so severe or damaging that a heart transplant is necessary

- Are categorized as acyanotic or cyanotic

Acyanotic Defects

Cardiac defects in which only, or predominantly, oxygenated blood enters the arterial circulation. The pressure on the left side of the heart is higher and allows the flow of blood to be shunted from the left to the right chambers. Cardiomegaly and pulmonary artery hypertrophy are commonly seen with this type of defect. The more commonly seen acyanotic defects include:

Atrial Septal Defect (ASD)

a. **Description** - The presence of an opening in the atrial septum. It may be due to the failure of the foramen ovale to close. Defects in this region of the atrial septum account for 9-10% of all lesions. Blood flows across the defect from left (high pressure) to right (low pressure) and causes increased pulmonary blood flow. The increased volume and workload result in right-sided hypertrophy and possibly mild to moderate pulmonary edema. This defect is seen more frequently in females.

b. **Signs and Symptoms** - Usually asymptomatic; may have audible systolic ejection murmur at left sternal border; mild exercise intolerance; mild to moderate cardiomegaly with pulmonary vascular disease gradually increasing

c. **Diagnostic Procedures** - ECG may reveal atrial arrhythmias (prolonged P-R interval); CXR reveals pulmonary vasculature, prominent pulmonary artery and right ventricle and atrium; echocardiogram reveals abnormal septal motion, allows for visualization of

ASD; angiography shows ASD; cardiac catherization reveals increased O_2 saturations in right atrium

d. Medical Interventions

- **Medications** - Administer digitalis and diuretics if right or left
  ventricular failure occur; administer antibiotics postoperatively.
- **Treatments** - May close spontaneously; monitor for signs of complications.
- **Surgery** - Surgical repair is performed only if defect is large or
  causing symptoms in boys and should always be repaired in girls
  due to the high risk of paradoxical emboli in pregnancy.

e. Nursing Interventions
  *See page 40.

f. Potential Complications - In adulthood: atrial arrhythmias, emboli,
  heart failure, left ventricular failure if uncorrected

Coarctation of the Aorta

a. Description - The presence of a narrowing anywhere along the aortic
  arch. This narrowing causes decreased blood flow distal to the structure, and the back up of blood flow in the heart. This defect is seen
  more frequently in males.

b. Signs and Symptoms - Usually depend upon severity; may
  experience hypertension in arterial branches proximal to the defect
  and hypotension distal to the defect; may be asymptomatic until
  adolescence if narrowing of area is mild; may have systolic murmur
  audible on back near left upper side; may have discrepancy in
  femoral pulses

c. Diagnostic Procedures- X-ray notes enlargement in portion of aorta
  proximal to stricture, cardiomegaly, and pulmonary edema; cardiac
  catheterization demonstrates location of defect; echocardiogram allows for visualization of defect

d. Medical Interventions

- **Medications** - Administer digitalis, dopamine, diuretics, oxygen,
  prostaglandin E (in newborns to keep ductus arteriosus open)
- **Treatment** - Provide fluid monitoring, renal monitoring, and rest;
  treatment for congestive heart failure may be required
- **Surgery** - Surgical repair to resect area and reanastomosis may
  be necessary sometime in childhood (subclavian flap aortoplasty)

e. Nursing Interventions

  *See page 40.

f. Potential Complications - Death from heart failure and renal shut-
  down preoperatively, infective endocarditis, renal failure postoperatively, recoarctation, death

Endocardial Cushion Defect - (Complete)

a. **Description** - The presence of a defect in the atrial septum and septal leaflets of the tricuspid and mitral valves. This results from failure to develop during the embryonic period. It presents as a wide spectrum of minor to major atrioventricular (AV) canals. With a complete defect, the patient has incomplete formation of mitral valve and tricuspid valves, ASD, and high ventricular septal defect. Blood flows through this opening and causes a mixing of oxygenated and un-oxygenated blood. It also causes increased pulmonary blood flow. The severity of the defect varies. This defect is seen equally in both sexes. A higher incidence is seen in children with Downs Syndrome.

b. **Signs and Symptoms** - May be asymptomatic at birth, may have audible systolic murmur and cyanosis upon exertion or crying, increased pulmonary congestion and edema, congestive heart failure, and delayed growth

c. **Diagnostic Procedures** - Diagnosed by physical findings; ECG reveals prolonged P-R interval; CXR reveals cardiomegaly and pulmonary vascular markings; echocardiogram allows for visualization of defects and shows communication between the 4 chambers of the heart

d. **Medical Interventions**
   - **Medications** - Administer digitalis, diuretics, antibiotics prophylactically
   - **Treatment** - Provide rest and monitor fluid status, prevent increased oxygen consumption.
   - **Surgery** - Surgical repair of the septum is performed and child may also require valve replacement or pulmonary artery banding, may be delayed until age 5 if child is essentially asymptomatic.

e. **Nursing Interventions**
   * See page 40.

f. **Potential Complications** - Heart failure, mitral regurgitation, congestive heart failure, complete heart block, arrhythmias postoperatively , death

Patent Ductus Arteriosus - (PDA)

a. **Description** - The presence of a passageway (ductus arteriosis) between the pulmonary and aortic circulation which persists after birth. This defect is caused by the failure of the fetal ductus arteriosis to close. The defect allows flow of blood from the aorta (high pressure) back into the pulmonary circulation (low pressure). It causes increased pulmonary blood flow. This defect often closes naturally by 6 months of age. The child may also have a VSD and/or coarctation of the aorta. This defect is seen more frequently in females and accounts for 10% of congenital heart defects.

    b. Signs and Symptoms - Typically present at birth; audible "washing machine" murmur at the left sternal border, may also have widened pulse pressures and bounding pulses; increased volume to the lungs may result in volume overload.

    c. Diagnostic Procedures - Diagnosed by physical findings; CXR may appear normal if defect is small or may reveal left-sided cardiomegaly if defect is large; echocardiogram allows for direct visualization of defect; ECG normal if defect small, but indicates left ventricular hypertrophy if defect is large

    d. Medical Interventions
- **Medications** - Administer Indomethacin
- **Treatment** - Monitor cardiac and pulmonary status, I&O
- **Surgery** - If asymptomatic, surgical repair is usually not utilized until the child becomes older (1-2 years). If systomatic (inability to wean from supplemental oxygen), PDA is ligated or banded.

    e. Nursing Interventions

      * See page 40.

    f. Potential Complications - Before surgery: pneumonia, pulmonary edema, congestive heart failure; postoperatively: infective endocarditis, pneumothorax, death

Pulmonary Stenosis - (PS)

    a. Description - A narrowing of one or more sites at the entrance of the pulmonary artery. This defect causes a resistance to the pulmonary artery, decreased pulmonary blood flow, a resistance to blood flow and, therefore, abnormally high right ventricular pressure and right ventricular hypertrophy.

    b. Signs and Symptoms - May be asymptomatic, findings depend upon the severity of the defect but may include a systolic ejection murmur audible with systolic thrill, complaint of dyspnea, and fatigue; may also be cyanotic and experience right ventricular failure and low cardiac output.

    c. Diagnostic Procedures - X-ray and echocardiogram reveal enlarged right ventricle; echocardiogram shows defect and thickened pulmonary valve; cardiac catheterization not necessary to confirm defect

    d. Medical Interventions
- **Medications** - Digitalis, diuretics, prophylactic antibiotics if valve involvement present
- **Treatment** - Balloon valvuloplasty during cardiac catheterization may be utilized to dilate area.
- **Surgery** - Surgical intervention is performed if symptoms are moderate to severe; surgeon may need to replace the pulmonic

valve if it is involved (pulmonic valvuloplasty or complete excision of dysplastic valve).

e. Nursing Interventions

*See page 40.

f. Potential Complications - Congestive heart failure, low cardiac output, infective endocarditis, death

Ventricular Septal Defect (VSD)

a. Description - VSD is the most commonly seen of the cardiac defects (comprises 20%). It is an opening between the right and left ventricles. It causes increased pulmonary blood flow. It may be associated with other defects or occur independently.

b. Signs and Symptoms - Usually asymptomatic, loud pansystolic murmur may be present; if large defect, may exhibit decreased exercise tolerance, increased respiratory infections, delayed growth and development, congestive heart failure, left ventricular hypertrophy and pulmonary edema

c. Diagnostic Procedures - Larger VSD defects are detected by CXR which shows enlarged left atria and ventricle; echocardiogram reveals size and location of defect.

d. Medical Interventions

- **Medications** - Administer digitalis, diuretics, and antibiotics prophylactically
- **Treatment** - Spontaneous closure may occur if small.
- **Surgery** - Treatment depends upon the severity of the defect. Surgical closure is performed if the VSD does not close spontaneously; if poor surgical risk, pulmonary artery banding may be done palliatively; recently, closure of defect is accomplished by placing occluding device into defect during cardiac catheterization

e. Nursing Interventions

* See page 40.

f. Potential Complications - Congestive heart failure, pulmonary edema, respiratory infections, altered growth and development, death

Cyanotic Defects

Cyanotic defects are defects in which unoxygenated blood mixes with some oxygenated blood in the heart. A large amount of unoxygenated blood then leaves the heart going into circulation. These defects cause the blood to flow from the right to the left side of the heart. More commonly seen cyanotic defects include:

Tetralogy of Fallot

   a. Description - This defect comprises 10% of all reported defects and is seen in both sexes. It causes decreased pulmonary blood flow and consists of 4 anomalies (each with varying severity):

   – Ventricular septal defect
   – Pulmonary stenosis
   – Overriding aorta
   – Right ventricular hypertrophy

   b. Signs and Symptoms - The predominate findings are cyanosis (degree depends upon severity of pulmonary stenosis), hypoxic spells after 2 months of age, pansystolic murmur, clubbing of fingers and toes (if defect continues long term without treatment); delay in growth and development; polycythemia; child will frequently take a squatting position after walking or playing to increase blood flow to the heart or may draw up the extremities when lying down.

   c. Diagnostic Procedures - Diagnosed by physical findings; ABGs reveal hypoxemia and acidosis; echocardiogram allows for visualization of defect; CXR shows right atrial and ventricular hypertrophy, normal left atrium and ventricle and small main pulmonary artery giving heart a boot-shaped appearance.

   d. Medical Interventions

   – **Medications** - Administer oxygen, digitalis, diuretics, and antibiotics prophylactically
   – **Treatment** - Limit activity, monitor I&O
   – **Surgery** - Surgical repair of the VSD and pulmonary stenosis is done according to severity of the symptoms (usually at 18 months). If underdeveloped pulmonary arteries are present, a systemic-to-pulmonary shunt is created (Blalock-Taussig procedure). There is a low mortality rate associated with this repair. Cardiac medications may be administered before surgery to treat symptoms and after surgery to enhance the function of the heart.

   e. Nursing Interventions

   * See page 40.

   f. Potential Complications - Postoperative bleeding, congestive heart failure, heart block, death

2. TRANSPOSITION OF THE GREAT VESSELS (TGV)

   a. Description - A defect in which the aorta arises from the right ventricle and the pulmonary artery arises from the left ventricle, i.e. the two great vessels are reversed. This reversal creates two independently functioning circulatory systems. The severity of the defect depends upon the amount of blood being mixed. Usually a patent foramen ovale and/or ventricular septal defect or PDA are present to maintain the infant's life after birth. The infant cannot survive unless these defects are present. This defect is seen more frequently in males and there may be a family history of diabetes.

b. **Signs and Symptoms** - Cardinal sign is severe cyanosis; audible murmur from the VSD and ASD, congestive heart failure develops shortly after birth; difficulty in feeding. Cyanosis and hypoxia increase as fetal structures (ductus arteriosis and foramen ovale) close.

c. **Diagnostic Procedures** - Diagnosed by physical findings; ABGs reveal hypoxemia and acidosis; labs reveal hypoglycemia, hypocalcemia, and polycythemia; CXR reveals cardiomegaly, egg-shaped heart silhouette; echocardiogram allows for visualization of defect

d. **Medical Interventions**
   - **Medications** - Administer prostaglandin (to keep foramen ovale open), digitalis, diuretics
   - **Treatment** - May be palliative or the defect may be corrected surgically; palliative treatment includes enlarging the other defects or making the necessary defects if not present (ASD or VSD); making a shunt to allow mixing of the blood thereby increasing oxygenated blood to flow into the circulation; correction metabolic acidosis, hypoglycemia, and hypocalcemia, administering oxygen
   - **Surgery** - Surgical correction usually takes place before 1 year of age.

e. **Nursing Interventions**
   * See page 40.

f. **Potential Complications** - Arrhythmias, pulmonary vascular obstructive disease, residual shunting, death

3. NURSING INTERVENTIONS FOR CONGENITAL DEFECTS

a. **Assessment and Actions**
   - Be alert to signs and symptoms that may indicate a possible defect and make a thorough assessment of the infant/child using inspection, auscultation, and palpation.
   - Assess child's vital signs, weight, hydration status, activity level, color, respiratory efforts, nutritional status, and activity level of comfort.
   - Monitor cardiac functioning (vital signs, EKG, respiratory efforts, skin color and temperature, I&O) preoperatively.
   - Postoperatively monitor level of comfort and provide method of reducing discomfort.
   - Assess for signs indicating potential complications.

b. **Teaching**
   - Assess family and child's level of understanding.
   - Explain diagnosis to child and family.

- Prepare the child and family for procedures and treatments by explaining the information clearly, allowing time for questions, and utilizing pictures or written information as indicated.
- Inform family, as indicated, if child may be at higher risk for developing complications which may include:
  - Infection or pain postprocedure and/or postoperatively
  - Congestive heart failure
  - Bacterial endocarditis
- Inform parents of special limitations of child's activity according to defect and suggest ways to enhance growth and development.
- Teach family about medications child will receive before and after corrective repair. Include name of drug, dose, times of administration, side effects, adverse reactions, and long term side effects.
- Prepare for discharge by teaching parents: how to care for child after procedures or surgery; what activity limitations are indicated; signs and symptoms that require further medical attention; and, provide phone numbers if questions or problems arise.

c. Emotional Care
- Be prepared to assist the family in the grieving process.
- Acknowledge parental concerns and concerns of the child.
- Allow child to voice concerns and ask questions.
- Promote growth and development while hospitalized.
- Provide support to family and child.
- Provide support group information to family.

Acquired Heart Defects

Acquired heart defects include those diseases which are caused by:
1). A secondary defect to an injured or defective heart
2). A new disease
3). Unknown causes

1. BACTERIAL ENDOCARDITIS (BE)

a. **Description** - An infection of the heart valves and inner lining of the heart valves which usually occurs in children with congenital cardiac defects, cardiac injuries or cardiac repairs.

b. **Signs and Symptoms** - Audible new murmur, anorexia, malaise, intermittent low grade fever, weight loss, petechiae, splinter hemorrhaging

c. **Diagnostic Procedures** - Diagnosed by history of previous cardiac defect or surgery; physical findings; CBC reveals anemia; presence of increased ESR; microscopic hematuria; echocardiogram reveals vegetative growth; blood cultures are positive for the organism.

d. **Medical Interventions**
  - **Medications** - Administer penicillin G or oxacillin, IV gentamicin, or IM streptomycin for 4-6 weeks
  - **Treatment** - Limit activity
  - **Surgery** - Valve replacement may be necessary if congestive heart failure develops, valve malfunctions, infection persists or relapse occurs.

e. **Nursing Interventions**
  - **Assessment and Actions**
    • Be alert to signs and symptoms of disorder.
    • Preoperatively and postoperatively assess vital signs, I&O, skin temperature and color, level of comfort.
    • Assess for signs indicating potential complications.
  - **Teaching**
    • Instruct patient and family on methods of prevention via prophylactic treatment to high risk candidates especially prior to visiting the dentist.
    • Explain diagnosis to parent and child.
    • Explain treatment regimen, length and purpose.
    • Inform parents of signs and symptoms and who to contact.
    • Teach parents and child about medication prescribed (drug, dose, route, time and side effects).
  - **Emotional Care**
    • Discuss concerns that family and child have
    • Provide support to family and child

f. **Potential Complications** - Persistent infection, congestive heart failure, death

2. **CONGESTIVE HEART FAILURE (CHF)**
  a. **Description** - A type of cardiac malfunction which causes a diminished amount of blood to be ejected into the systemic circulation. CHF usually does not occur in children unless another cardiac disorder precedes it. It may be either predominantly right-sided or left-sided failure of the heart muscle.
  b. **Signs and Symptoms** - Dyspnea, fatigue, weakness, poor feeding and growth, sweating, coughing, pallor, cyanosis, cardiomegaly, tachycardia, tachypnea, and edema
  c. **Diagnostic Procedures** - Diagnosed by physical findings, CXR reveals cardiomegaly; echocardiogram assists with determining cause
  d. **Medical Interventions**
    - **Medications** - Administer oxygen, sedation (morphine), diuretics and digoxin

- **Treatment** - Correct underlying cause and improve heart function and tissue oxygenation; restrict sodium and fluid intake; monitor I&O
- **Surgery** - Unnecessary unless to correct underlying cause.

e. **Nursing Interventions**
  - **Assessment and Actions**
    - Be alert for signs and symptoms of CHF.
    - If hospitalized, monitor vital signs, lung sounds, edema, daily weight, and assess nutritional status.
    - Administer medications on schedule.
    - Draw digoxin levels as ordered noting results.
    - Observe signs of Digoxin toxicity (changes in ECG).
    - Provide skin care and frequently turn patient to prevent skin breakdown.
    - Place in cardiac chair or infant chair.
    - Assess for signs indicating potential complications.
  - **Teaching**
    - Discuss diagnosis and treatment plan with parent and child
    - Instruct parent and child on medication prescribed (drug, dose, route, time, and side effects).
    - Inform parents and child of signs of digitalis toxicity. Signs and symptoms include nausea, vomiting, anorexia, and bradycardia. Dysrhythmias may also occur in severe cases.
    - Encourage parents to have child rest as much as possible to decrease the heart's workload.
    - Emphasize importance of adequate nutritional intake for child.
  - **Emotional Care**
    - Discuss impact disease has had on child and family
    - Provide support to family and child
    - Provide support group information to family

f. **Potential Complications** - Digoxin toxicity, skin breakdown, respiratory infections, death

3. RHEUMATIC FEVER (ACUTE)

a. **Description** - Rheumatic fever is an inflammatory disease which can affect many body systems including the heart, joints, and subcutaneous tissue. It is thought to commonly follow an upper respiratory infection (Group A streptococci). It may occur at any age but primarily affects middle to late childhood.

b. Signs and Symptoms
- **Findings include**:
  - Carditis with accompanying murmur, cardiomegaly, tachycardia, CHF, Aschoff bodies (lesions that cause scarring and fibrosis of the cusps of the valves)
  - Polyarthritis - redness, swelling, pain, heat in multiple joints
  - Chorea (involuntary movements)
  - Erythema marginatum (macular rash on trunk and extremities)
  - Subcutaneous nodules in joints, scalp and spine
  - Other nonspecific findings which may include anorexia, low-grade fever, and fatigue.

c. Diagnostic Procedures - Diagnosis is made by utilizing Jones criteria and is positive for the disease if there is evidence of two major or one major and two minor criteria with positive ASO titer.

Jones Criteria:

Major Manifestations
- Polyarthritis
- Carditis
- Chorea
- Erythema marginatum
- Elevated ESR + CRP
- Subcutaneous nodules

Minor Manifestations
- Fever
- Arthralgia
- History of RF or RHD
- Acute phase reactants
- Prolonged P-R interval

d. Medical Interventions
- **Medications** - Administer benzathine penicillin G, anti-inflammatories (prednisone) and salicylates (to reduce the inflammation); begin prophylactic antibiotic therapy once inflammation is resolved; phenobarbital, chlorpromazine or diazepam may be used to treat chorea
- **Treatment** - Keep patient on bedrest to prevent stress and injury to the joints and heart.
- **Surgery** - Unnecessary

e. Nursing Interventions
- **Assessment and Actions**
  - Be alert to signs and symptoms which may indicate rheumatic fever.
  - Provide method of reducing discomfort (warm compresses, positioning, analgesics, antipyretics).
  - Assess for signs indicating potential complications.
- **Teaching**
  - Assist family in understanding disease process and cause.

- Explain importance of keeping child on bedrest until disease is resolved.
- Encourage family to provide adequate nutrition to promote healing during active disease state.
- Emphasize importance of compliance with long-term prophylaxis and medication administration.
- Teach parents and child about medication prescribed (drug, dose, route, time and side effects).

– **Emotional Care**
  - Provide support to parent and child.
  - Promote growth and development.
  - Provide support to family and child.
  - Provide support group information to family.

f. **Potential Complications** - Permanent cardiac damage to valves

5

GASTROINTESTINAL DISORDERS

I.   General Concepts

- Gastrointestinal (GI) disorders may occur anywhere along the GI tract.

- The GI system functions to provide nutrient ingestion, absorption, and elimination by mechanical and chemical breakdown.

- At birth the GI system is immature and continues to grow in size and functioning ability until it reaches its mature size and functioning level during the schoolage years.

- GI disorders may be congenital, acquired, acute or chronic.

- GI disorders are one of the most frequently seen abnormalities in childhood and are frequently managed at home.

- Dehydration from severe vomiting or diarrhea poses a serious threat and can occur rapidly.

- Hospital discharge planning is important for the nurse to consider to enhance compliance with the treatment regimen and to maintain the child in a normal home environment.

II. Specific Gastrointestinal Disorders

Congenital Disorders

1. CLEFT LIP/PALATE

a. **Description** - Malformation of the lip, maxilla, soft and/or hard palate. It may involve the lip and/or palate and may be unilateral or bilateral.

b. **Signs and Symptoms** - Lack of fusion of lip and/or soft or hard palate upon inspection

c. **Diagnostic Procedures** - Diagnosed by characteristic physical findings

d. **Medical Interventions**
   - **Medications** - Administer antibiotics postoperatively.
   - **Treatments** - Based on defect; may also have increased frequency of otitis media which should be monitored
   - **Surgery**
     * *Cleft lip* - closure of lip(s) with sutures or reconstruction (when child is 1-2 months); sutures secured with Logan bow
     * *Cleft palate* - surgical closure after lip repair (when child is 4-18 months of age); may be done in stages

e. **Nursing Interventions**
   - **Assessment and Actions**
     * Assess newborn for defect.
     * Provide adequate nutrition by using special nipples (Lamb's nipple or special nurser).
     * Prevent aspiration by holding infant upright during feedings and aspirating excess mucous or formula from nose.
     * Monitor hydration status and weight before discharged.
     * Assist with organizing other healthcare professionals (speech therapy, audiology, nutritionist, occupational therapists, dentists).
     * Postoperatively - If lip repair: maintain Logan bow in place to reduce sutureline tension, restrain child if necessary, keep surgical area clean, observe for signs of infection, provide comfort measures, prevent vigorous sucking until lip area healed, promote infant stimulation and interaction with parents. If palate repair: prevent any sharp object from going into mouth until area healed; restrain arms unless infant is attended by an adult.
     * Assess for signs indicating potential complications.
   - **Teaching**
     * Explain defect, plan of treatment and time of typical surgical repair.
     * Discuss potential need for dental prosthetic devices before and after surgery and necessity of good dental hygiene.

- Instruct parents on method of feeding, amount of formula, and length of time to allow infant to feed before and after surgery.
- Teach parent how to use bulb syringe and tube feeding if necessary.

- **Emotional Care**
  - Facilitate bonding following birth.
  - Determine parents' response to infant and provide support.
  - Provide support to family.
  - Provide support group information to family.
- **Potential Complications** - Minor physical deformity or scarring, chronic otitis media, speech deficits, difficulty in parents bonding with child

2. CONGENITAL DIAPHRAGMATIC HERNIA

a. **Description** - The incomplete formation of the diaphragm during fetal development (most often resulting from the failure of the Foramen of Bochdalek to close) allowing the abdominal contents to herniate through a diaphragmatic hole into the pleural cavity. It most commonly occurs on the left side, and it requires emergency surgery. There is a high mortality rate if symptoms are present at birth.

b. **Signs and Symptoms** - Dyspnea, respiratory distress shortly after birth, flattened (scaphoid) abdominal appearance, vomiting, full or barrel chest appearance, difficulty feeding, absence of breath sounds on affected side of chest

c. **Diagnostic Procedures** - X-ray reveals air filled loops of bowel or gastric bubble in thoracic space of affected side.

d. **Medical Interventions**
   - **Medications** - Administer antibiotics, vasopressors, volume expanders, sedation, and pharmacologic paralyzing agents postoperatively
   - **Treatments** - Maintain pulmonary function before and after surgery, do NOT face bag infant, place Salem sump to decompress GI tract, elevate head of bed to downward displace abdominal contents from chest, ECG and echocardiogram ordered to rule out cardiac involvement (hypoplastic left heart syndrome), extracorporeal membrane oxygenation (ECMO) immediately following delivery or during immediate postoperative period (these infants have a high mortality and morbidity rate related to persistent pulmonary hypertension)
   - **Surgery** - Surgical repair of defect is essential and is performed immediately after diagnosis is made.

e. **Nursing Interventions**
   - **Assessment and Actions**
     - Assess newborn for signs of defect.

- Preoperatively keep infant in high Fowler's position, place NG tube to prevent aspiration, administer oxygen as ordered, administer IV fluids, monitor for signs of severe respiratory distress
- Postoperatively assess respiratory status, hydration status, bowel sounds, position infant in high Fowler's, administer sedations and other medications as ordered
- Assess for signs indicating potential complications.

- **Teaching**
  - Explain defect, diagnostic procedures and treatment to parents, allowing time for questions.
  - Inform parents of how infant will appear postoperatively.

- **Emotional Care**
  - Allow parents to interact and bond with child as soon as possible.
  - Provide support to family.

f. **Potential Complications** - Respiratory failure, circulatory problems before and after surgery, infection, Broncopulmonary Dysplasia (BPD - related to prolonged mechanical ventilation and persistent pulmonary hypertension), heart failure, death

3. IMPERFORATE ANUS

a. **Description** - An abnormality in the formation of the anorectal area. The malformation may be classified as low, intermediate or high anomaly. Other defects are often present.

b. **Signs and Symptoms** - Depends upon location and type of defect: inability to pass stool, no visible anal opening, constipation and difficulty
stooling, ribbon-like bowel movements, increased abdominal girth, inability or difficulty in taking rectal temperature

c. **Diagnostic Procedures** - Visual inspection, digital examination, and x-ray

d. **Medical Interventions**
  - **Medications** - Administer antibiotics postoperatively.
  - **Treatments** - Depend upon location and severity of defect, but if mild includes digital or instrumental dilatation of anal opening
  - **Surgery** - Repair or reconstruction of anal opening or anastomosis of section of bowel not joined, placement of temporary or permanent colostomy may be required

e. **Nursing Interventions**
  - **Assessment and Actions**
    - Be alert to signs and symptoms of disorder.
    - Monitor stooling pattern before and after treatment/surgery.

- Postoperatively monitor vital signs, surgical site, level of comfort, and provide method of pain control.
- Assist with organizing home care service.
- Assess for signs indicating potential complications.

- **Teaching**
  - Explain diagnosis to parents and discuss treatment regimen.
  - Teach parents how to digitally dilate area, if ordered.
  - Discuss with parents and child what to expect before and after surgery.
  - Teach parents colostomy and skin care prior to discharge, if needed.
  - Provide parents with anticipatory guidance and potential difficulty with toilet training if sphincter involved.
  - Teach bowel training regimen.

- **Emotional Care**
  - Provide support to family.
  - Provide support group information to family.

f. **Potential Complications** - Loss of bowel control, infection, perforation, permanent ostomy, skin breakdown.

4. OMPHALOCELE/GASTROSCHISIS

a. **Description** - A malformation of the abdominal wall allowing intestinal contents to protrude either through the umbilical cord (omphalocele) or through the abdominal wall not involving the umbilical cord (gastroschisis). It is often associated with other anomalies.

b. **Signs and Symptoms** - Visible defect at birth; abdominal contents protruding through abdominal wall

c. **Diagnostic Procedures** - Diagnosed upon inspection

d. **Medical Interventions**
   - **Medications** - Administer broad spectrum antibiotics, sedation, analgesics postoperatively
   - **Treatments** - Maintain protective covering over sac preoperatively.
   - **Surgery** - Correct by returning abdominal contents to abdominal wall (either by gravity or surgical reduction).

e. **Nursing Interventions**
   - **Assessment and Actions**
     - Be alert to signs of defect in newborn (defect may be detected on ultrasound prior to delivery).
     - Postoperatively monitor vital signs, respiratory status, venous return, level of comfort; observe for signs of infection or rupture, assess bowel sounds.

- Preoperatively maintain moist and sterile dressing on pouch, prevent rupture of soc; monitor vital signs, hydration, and temperature; position child supine, place NG tube and IV line.
- Provide method for reducing discomfort.
- Assess for signs indicating potential complications.
  - **Teaching**
    - Explain defect to parents and treatment regimen, allowing for questions.
    - Teach parents incision care and care of child at home.
  - **Emotional Care**
    - Encourage bonding of parents with infant as soon as possible.
    - Provide support to family.
  f. **Potential Complications** - Rupture of sac prior to repair, infection, necrosis of bowel, obstruction, respiratory compromise postoperatively

5. **PYLORIC STENOSIS**
   a. **Description**-The hypertrophy of the pyloric sphincter causing a narrowing of the normal passageway between the stomach and small intestines. It is most frequently congenital but may also be acquired and is seen in male infants more often.

   b. **Signs and Symptoms** - Projectile vomiting after feeding during first or second week of life; infant appears well and hungry but exhibits poor weight gain, distended abdomen with palpable olive-size mass in right upper quadrant, also exhibits visible peristaltic activity in abdomen, dehydration

   c. **Diagnostic Procedures** - Diagnosed by characteristic history, physical inspection, ability to palpate olive-sized mass in right upper quadrant; X-ray after barium ingestion reveals stenosis (railroad track sign)

   d. **Medical Interventions**
      - **Medications** - Administer antibiotics and analgesics postoperatively
      - **Treatments** - Place NG tube, correct dehydration and electrolyte imbalance
      - **Surgery** - Perform pyloromyotomy within 24 hours of diagnosis

   e. **Nursing Interventions**
      - **Assessment and Actions**
        - Be alert to signs and symptoms that indicate disorder.
        - Preoperatively maintain hydration, fluid and electrolyte balance and keep infant NPO.
        - Postoperatively monitor vital signs, hydration status, monitor bowel sounds and for signs of infection.
        - Provide methods for reducing discomfort postoperatively.

- **Teaching**
  - Explain defect and treatment to parents.
  - Discuss length of hospitalization (usually 3-4 days).
  - Teach care of incision.
- **Emotional Care**
  - Continue to promote bonding between infant and parents.
  - Provide support to parents.

f. Potential Complications - Infection, fluid and electrolyte imbalance, dehydration, shock (prognosis is good)

6. TRACHEOESOPHAGEAL FISTULA (TEF)

a. Description - A malformation of the esophagus and/or tracheal passageway. It may involve diversion of the esophageal contents into a blind sac, into the trachea, or into the trachea then stomach or lungs. It can be life threatening.

b. Signs and Symptoms - Difficulty feeding, coughing, choking, frequent regurgitation; becomes cyanotic during feedings; excessive drooling; typically has immediate onset of respiratory distress

c. Diagnostic Procedures - Diagnosed by inability to pass NG/OG catheter or by NG/OG tube curling back into mouth; fluoroscopic visualization of passing catheter shows obstruction or abnormal passageway; x-ray with radiopaque catheter shows dilated upper esophageal pouch

d. Medical Interventions

- **Medications** - Administer antibiotics prophylactically and postoperatively; sedation and analgesics postoperatively.
- **Treatments** - Provide IV hydration and nutrition, prevent aspiration, place Salem sump tube to low intermittent suction, monitor for pulmonary infections.
- **Surgery** - Requires surgical dilatation, anastamosis of esophageal passageway with placement of temporary gastrostomy or cervical esophagosotomy

e. Nursing Interventions

- **Assessment and Actions**
  - Be alert to signs and symptoms that indicate disorder.
  - Preoperatively monitor vital signs, hydration status, respiratory function, keep NPO, prevent aspiration, keep infant comfortable, have suction equipment available, try to prevent excessive crying, keep head of bed elevated.
  - Postoperatively monitor vital signs, hydration status, I&O, respiratory status, incision, observe for signs of infection or perforation.
  - Provide means for reducing discomfort.
  - Assess for signs indicating potential complications.

- **Teaching**
  - Explain diagnosis to parents and explain treatment regimen
  - Instruct parents on suctioning, feeding technique, signs of respiratory difficulty if treatment is delayed or to be done in stages.
  - Teach ostomy care and how to feed child through esophagostomy if surgical correction is to be performed.
  - Teach parents how to use bulb syringe.
- **Emotional Care**
  - Encourage parents to care for infant to promote bonding.
  - Provide support to family.
  - Provide support group information to family.

f. **Potential Complications** - Aspiration, pneumonia, dehydration, infection, esophageal strictures, death from aspiration or lack of patency of trachea to lungs

Acquired Disorders

1. APPENDICITIS (ACUTE)

a. **Description** - A swelling or inflammation of the appendix (vermiform appendix). It may lead to perforation and peritonitis if it is left untreated. It occurs more commonly in the school-age child.

b. **Signs and Symptoms** - Fever, abdominal tenderness at McBurney's point, rebound tenderness in lower right abdomen, diminished bowel sounds, vomiting, legs drawn up to chest while lying down

c. **Diagnostic Procedures** - Elevated WBC present, x-ray reveals right curve of spine due to muscle spasm, fecalith may be visible. If perforation has occurred, free peritoneal fluid is visible on x-ray.

d. **Medical Interventions**
  - **Medications** - Administer antibiotics postoperatively and preoperatively if rupture occurred, analgesics post operatively
  - **Treatments** - Monitor I&O and discomfort pre and postoperatively.
  - **Surgery** - Surgical removal (appendectomy) is necessary to prevent rupture and potential peritonitis; if rupture occurs, surgical correction must be performed immediately.

e. **Nursing Interventions**
  - **Assessment and Actions**
    - Be alert to signs and symptoms that indicate disorder.
    - Preoperatively observe for signs of rupture: sudden absence of pain and change in vital signs indicating sepsis or shock.
    - Assess for level of comfort and provide method for reducing discomfort before, during and after surgery.

- Postoperatively assess vital signs, bowel sounds, fluid and electrolyte status; position in Semi Fowler's or on right side, monitor for signs of infection.
- Assess for signs indicating potential complications.

 — Teaching
- Explain procedures and surgical interventions to parents and child.
- Discuss presence and purpose of postoperative equipment and treatment (penrose drain, NG tube, I.V. fluids, NPO status).
- Teach parents about medications prescribed (drug, dose, route, time, and side effects).

 — Emotional Care
- Provide support to family and child.
- Encourage parent to stay with child if possible.

f. Potential Complications - Preoperatively, if rupture occurs, peritonitis, shock; postoperatively, infection.

2. CELIAC DISEASE (GLUTEN-SENSITIVE ENTEROPATHY)

a. Description - The inability of the bowel to tolerate gluten (protein found in oats, rye, barley and wheat). This intolerance causes problems with absorption of fats, carbohydrates, proteins, vitamins D, B12, and K, calcium, iron, and folic acid in the bowel. It is rarely seen in Blacks and Asians. Signs and symptoms typically appear before 2 years of age or after age 5.

b. Signs and Symptoms - Diarrhea, constipation, vomiting, abdominal tenderness and distension, anemia, failure to gain weight, irritability, apathy, loss of subcutaneous fat, muscle wasting, dependent edema in lower extremities; Celiac crisis-bulky, greasy, frothy, pale, foul smelling stools (steatorrhea), smooth tongue, atrophy in extremities and buttocks, and edema

c. Diagnostic Procedures - Stool analysis reveals steatorrhea, small bowel biopsy reveals alteration in villi, D-xylose absorption test and lactose H2 breath test are abnormal; sweat chloride test performed to rule out cystic fibrosis

d. Medical Interventions

 — Medications - Administer corticosteroid (prn), vitamin and mineral supplements, TPN if severely malnourished
 — Treatments - Life-long dietary restriction of gluten-containing products (rye, oats, barley)
 — Surgery - Unnecessary

e. Nursing Interventions

 — Assessment and Actions
- Be alert for signs and symptoms.
- Monitor child's growth and development

- Assess for signs indicating potential complications.
  - **Teaching**
    - Explain diagnosis and implications of treatment regimen to parents and child.
    - Instruct parents on gluten-free diet--no ingestion of oats, wheat, rye, and barley and importance of adherence throughout child's life.
    - Teach parents and child causes of celiac crisis: poor diet adherence, stress, and infection; discuss potential life-threatening nature of crisis (may cause dehydration and metabolic acidosis).
  - **Emotional Care**
    - Provide support to family and child.
    - Discuss how disease is impacting child and family's lifestyle.
    - Provide support group information to family.
  - f. **Potential Complications** - If diet not adhered to relapse may occur; long-term noncompliance may lead to anemia, growth retardation, osteomalacia, GI problems (change in mucosal lining, potential increase in incidence of cancer); celiac crisis.

3. **GASTROENTERITIS/DIARRHEA (ACUTE)**

   a. **Description** - An inflammation of the stomach and intestines which may be acute or chronic and causes diarrhea. It may be caused by a variety of organisms, nutritional intake, anatomical disturbance, allergies, disease processes, toxic ingestion, or neoplastic abnormalities. It is frequently seen in the pediatric population.

   b. **Signs and Symptoms** - Depend upon severity, causative factor, duration and age of child; presence of frequent diarrheal episodes, dehydration, fluid and electrolyte disturbances; may lead to shock if severe

   c. **Diagnostic Procedures** - Diagnostic tests vary with causative factors; stool cultures determine if ova or parasites, blood, mucous, bacteria present; dietary intake assessment (determines if lactose intolerance present), x-rays check for obstruction or abnormality, blood cultures used to determine if organisms present; may also screen for toxic ingestion.

   d. **Medical Interventions**
      - **Medications** - Administer antibiotics (if caused by organisms), antispasmodics, or bismuth subsalicylate
      - **Treatments** - Discontinue foods and fluids containing lactose; mild and moderate dehydration may be treated at home by offering child oral glucose-electrolyte fluids (ex: Pedialyte); if dehydration is severe, IV fluids are necessary to achieve fluid and electrolyte balance; may require a change in diet (if allergic use

BRATS diet: bananas, rice, applesauce, toast, saltines) until episode resolved
  - **Surgery** - Unnecessary unless mass or defect noted
- **e. Nursing Interventions**
  - **Assessment and Actions**
    - Be alert to signs and symptoms that indicate disorder.
    - Assist with determining level of dehydration (mild, moderate, severe) and causative factor.
    - Provide care according to severity of dehydration and cause:
      - **Mild and moderate** - Instruct parents on home care on increasing fluids, changing type of diet and/or medication therapy, and inform parents to call if signs of dehydration and diarrhea persist.
      - **Severe** - Hospitalization required, monitor weight, I&O, vital signs, maintain IV site; monitor and record stools (frequency, consistency, amount, appearance), provide method for reducing discomfort and prevent perineal skin breakdown; isolation and enteric precautions may be necessary, depending upon the causative factor
    - Provide progressive diet as ordered (liquids, to soft diet, to full diet).
    - Assess for signs indicating potential complications.
  - **Teaching**
    - Explain diagnosis to parent and child.
    - Instruct parent if child is to be cared for at home how to administer a progressive diet: liquids to soft to full diet or if dietary cause to remove source of irritant from child's diet.
    - Teach parent how to prevent skin breakdown of the buttocks and perineal area and prevent secondary infections.
    - Instruct parent to observe for signs of severe dehydration and when to notify the physician if symptoms worsen.
  - **Emotional Care**
    - Provide support to family and child.
- **f. Potential Complications** - Skin breakdown, metabolic acidosis, severe dehydration may cause shock and death if left untreated

4. GASTROESOPHAGEAL REFLUX

- **a. Description** - The presence of an abnormality in the cardiac sphincter allowing the stomach contents to flow back into the esophagus. It is frequently seen in infants (particularly preterm) until sphincter control is achieved.

- **b. Signs and Symptoms** - Frequent, nonforceful vomiting especially after feedings, failure to thrive, esophagitis with bleeding noted in area, cyanosis, apnea, aspiration pneumonia, and choking

c. **Diagnostic Procedures** - Diagnosed by characteristic history and physical; barium esophagram reveals reflux, esophageal manometry assesses motility and lower esophageal sphincter pressure, pH probe placed anterior to sphincter indicates higher pH in esophagus

d. **Medical Interventions**
   - **Medications** - Administer bethanecol or metaclopromide, antacids, cimetidine (may be required)
   - **Treatments** - If weight loss is not occurring in infancy, then treatment is unnecessary; if Failure to Thrive (FTT) or apparent weight loss present, encourage parent to feed child in upright position, include cereal in formula.
   - **Surgery** - Surgical correction may be necessary if severe reflux present (Nissen fundoplication).

e. **Nursing Interventions**
   - **Assessment and Actions**
     - Be alert to signs that indicate disorder.
     - Monitor child's weight, I & O; measure amount, frequency, contents and time of vomiting.
     - Maintain reflux precautions (place supine and sitting upright or prone with elevated head of bed on slant board or with harness).
     - Provide method of reducing discomfort postoperatively.
     - Assess for signs indicating potential complications.
   - **Teaching**
     - Inform parents of diagnosis and treatment regimen.
     - Teach parents how to feed infant: offer small amounts of fluid to infant with infant in an upright position, burp frequently, after feeding hold infant in upright position or place infant prone with head of bed elevated (30 degrees).
     - Teach parents about medications prescribed (drug, dose, route, time, and side effects).
     - Teach parents how to use a bulb syringe.
   - **Emotional Care**
     - Prepare parents emotionally for child's surgery if required.
     - Provide support to family.

f. **Potential Complications** - Aspiration, anemia (if blood loss present), esophageal strictures, insufficient weight gain, apnea

5. **HIRSCHSPRUNG DISEASE (CONGENITAL AGANGLIONIC MEGACOLON)**

a. **Description** - A congenital abnormality in motility of a portion of the intestine causing an obstruction. It is due to an irregularity in innervation of bowel in which a segment is aganglionic and lacks peristalsis.

The colon proximal to the defect enlarges due to lack of peristalsis in the affected area of the colon.

b. Signs and Symptoms - Newborn's inability to pass meconium within first 24-48 hours, stool absent on rectal examination, increasing abdominal girth, bile-stained emesis, irritability, reluctance to feed, FTT, vomiting, constipation, explosive diarrhea. Childhood symptoms include abdominal firmness and distension, thin, foul-smelling ribbon-like bowel movements, constipation, poor weight gain

c. Diagnostic Procedures - X-ray demonstrates dilated loops of intestine in absence of rectal air; barium enema reveals narrowed segment of bowel; rectal manometry reveals absence of relaxation of internal sphincter; rectal biopsy confirms diagnosis

d. Medical Interventions
- **Medications** - Administer antibiotics postoperatively.
- **Treatments** - Enema therapy may be sufficient; place NG tube and rehydrate.
- **Surgery** - Correct by removing defective bowel, may be accompanied by temporary colostomy placement, rarely removal of entire colon and placement of permanent ileostomy.

e. Nursing Interventions
- **Assessment and Actions**
  - Be alert to signs and symptoms indicating disorder.
  - Monitor child's weight, I&O, fluid and electrolyte status, and abdominal girth.
  - Postoperatively keep child NPO, assess vital signs and for signs of infection, maintain hydration and assess bowel sounds, observe for signs of peritonitis or perforation of bowel, provide method for reducing discomfort.
  - Assist with establishing home care.
  - Assess for signs indicating potential complications.
- **Teaching**
  - Explain disorder and treatment regimen to parents.
  - If enema therapy is ordered instruct parents on how to administer, amount to instill, and importance of using normal saline solution.
  - Teach parents how to care for colostomy, obtain return demonstration and discuss nutritional needs before discharge.
- **Emotional Care**
  - Promote growth and development.
  - Provide support to family and child.
  - Provide support group information to family.

f. Potential Complications - Perforation and sepsis, peritonitis, poor bowel control, alteration in bonding, altered body image (child), persistent diarrhea, overflow incontinence, death

6. INFLAMMATORY BOWEL DISEASE
Ulcerative Colitis and Crohn's Disease*

a. **Descriptions**

- **Ulcerative Colitis** - An inflammatory disease of the mucosa and submucosa of the colon. It is typically seen in young adults, but may affect any age. It is more common in Caucasians, upper socioeconomic classes and Jewish populations (a familial tendency is suspected.) It is a chronic disorder with unknown etiology.

- **Crohn's Disease** - Transmural inflammation of the intestinal tract wall. Affected areas repeatedly become inflamed and heal, causing scarring and weakening of the intestine. It may affect any area from the mouth to the anus but most commonly affects the terminal ileum and anus. It is also more common among Caucasians and the Jewish population with a familial tendency noted. There are often several areas of intestine affected at the same time. It is also known as regional enteritis.

Both typically occur in the late schoolage or early adolescence age group.

b. **Signs and Symptoms** - Signs and symptoms are similar and include anemia, fever, dehydration, fluid and electrolyte disturbances, stools containing blood and/or mucous, delay in sexual maturation

COMPARISON OF SIGNS AND SYMPTOMS	
ULCERATIVE COLITIS	**CROHN'S DISEASE**
• Severe bloody diarrhea	• Frequent, watery diarrhea with or without blood
• Failure to thrive	• Abdominal pain (frequent)
• Abdominal pain	• Weight loss (severe)
• Weight loss (moderate)	• Moderate/severe anorexia
• Mild/moderate anorexia	• Severe growth failure
• Mild growth failure	• Rectal bleeding uncommon
• Rectal bleeding common	• Fissures/fistulas on barium enema
• Normal barium enema	

c. **Diagnostic Procedures** - (Both) stool analysis reveals blood and leukocytes; sigmoidoscopy reveals colitis; CBC may reveal anemia, leukocytosis, thrombocytosis, and increased ESR; barium enema reveals colitis; differentiated by intestinal biopsy; Ulcerative colitis reveals diffuse mucosal involvement with superficial ulcerations that are localized and contiguous; Crohn's disease reveals transmural lesions with deep ulcerations that are scattered throughout the intestine.

d. Medical Interventions
- **Medications** - Same for both disorders. Administer sulfasalazine, corticosteroids, antispasmodics, immunosuppressive agents, and total parenteral nutrition
- **Treatments** - Provide nutrition; total parenteral nutrition may be used to allow bowel to rest during exacerbations
- **Surgery** - Surgical removal of affected bowel (colectomy) may be cure for Ulcerative colitis; surgical resection for Crohn's disease is not beneficial due to the multiple patches present, surgical repair for complications of Crohn's disease may be needed and individual may need colostomy placement

e. Nursing Interventions - Same for both disorders
- **Assessment and Actions**
  - Be alert to signs and symptoms.
  - Postoperatively, monitor vital signs, abdominal girth, bowel sounds, suture line, and level of comfort.
  - Provide method for reducing discomfort.
  - Assess for signs indicating potential complications.
- **Teaching**
  - Explain diagnosis and treatment regimen to parent and child.
  - Instruct parents and child about diet therapy--high protein, low fat, low fiber, high calorie diet.
  - Inform parents and child of signs of exacerbations and remissions of disease and treatment required.
  - Teach parents and child about medication prescribed (drug, dose, route, time, and side effects).
  - Discuss care of colostomy or ileostomy, if necessary.
  - Emphasize need for follow-up care (increased incidence of colorectal cancer with each disorder).
- **Emotional Care**
  - Promote child's body image and self-esteem.
  - Encourage reducing stress as much as possible.
  - Provide support to family and child.
  - Provide support group information to family and child.

f. Potential Complications -(Same for both disorders) Perforation and sepsis; peritonitis; skin breakdown around ostomy; medications and stress level increased leading to exacerbations; malabsorption; growth retardation; at higher risk for colon cancer.

7. INTUSSUSCEPTION

a. **Description** - A telescoping of a portion of the intestine into itself causing an obstruction. It is the most common cause of intestinal obstruction in the first 2 years of life. The etiology is unknown. It is more common in children with gastroenteritis, cystic fibrosis, and celiac disease.

b. **Signs and Symptoms** - Paroxysmal, episodic acute pain in the abdomen, vomiting, stools change from normal to a "currant jelly" appearance with red tinge; a long, cylindrical mass may be palpable in affected area; may be life-threatening if bowel perforates or becomes necrotic

c. **Diagnostic Procedures** - Diagnosed by physical findings, x-ray reveals area affected, barium enema reveals affected area

d. **Medical Interventions**
   - **Medications** - Antibiotics may be given after reduction
   - **Treatments** - Hydrostatic reduction by barium enema; IV fluids
   - **Surgery** - If treatment is unsuccessful, then laparotomy and surgical reduction is necessary

e. **Nursing Interventions**
   - **Assessment and Actions**
     • Be alert to signs and symptoms.
     • Assess for signs of rupture or necrosis prior to correction of defect.
     • Post-correction care includes monitoring vital signs, assessing and monitoring bowel sounds and stooling, maintaining hydration status, providing method for reducing discomfort, monitoring for signs of infection and shock.
     • Assess for signs indicating potential complications.
   - **Teaching**
     • Inform parents about diagnosis and treatment regimen.
   - **Emotional Care**
     • Encourage parents to stay with child.
     • Provide support to family and child.

f. **Potential Complications** - Perforation, necrosis, peritonitis, reoccurrence of telescoping, death

8. VOMITING

a. **Description** - The expulsion of stomach or intestinal contents. It may be due to a variety of factors which include obstruction, infection, allergic reaction, toxins, tumors, and overfeeding.

b. **Signs and Symptoms** - Expulsion of stomach or intestinal contents containing either liquid or food particles; may vary in color, amount, frequency, forcefulness, odor and duration

c. **Diagnostic Procedures** - X-ray determines if obstruction is present; review of history determines if vomiting is due to other medications or possible exposure to poison

d. **Medical Interventions**
   - **Medications** - Administer antiemetic and IV fluids if dehydration is present.
   - **Treatment** - Treat cause, maintain hydration, monitor nutritional status, discontinue solid foods, administer clear fluids for 12-24 hours then utilize BRATS diet (bananas, rice, applesauce, toast, and saltines) and later advance to solids as tolerated.
   - **Surgery** - May be required if obstruction is the cause of disorder

e. **Nursing Interventions**
   - **Assessment and Actions**
     • Obtain thorough history of emetic episodes to include duration, frequency, color, odor, precipitating factors, alleviating factors.
     • Assess child's hydration status, vital signs, weight, level of consciousness, dietary intake.
     • Prevent aspiration by positioning child laterally.
     • If hospitalized, monitor vital signs, weight, hydration status, fluid and electrolytes; provide method of reducing discomfort, assess vomitus for blood, pH, and record amount, color and duration; maintain patent IV and advance diet as tolerated and ordered.
     • Assess for signs indicating potential complications.
   - **Teaching**
     • Discuss diagnosis and treatment regimen with parents.
     • Teach parents home management: diet progression from clear liquids to bland foods to full foods as tolerated; antiemetic administration; other treatments depending upon cause (antibiotics, identifying and removing stress or allergic sources)
   - **Emotional Care**
     • Provide support to family and child.

f. **Potential Complications** - Dehydration, fluid and electrolyte imbalance, shock

6

GENITOURINARY DISORDERS

I. General Concepts

- The genitourinary system functions to regulate the body's fluid and electrolyte status and remove metabolic waste products and toxins from the body.

- The kidneys and renal system of the infant are immature, resulting in inefficient regulation and concentration of solutes and waste products.

- Infants are unable to concentrate urine until the age of one year, therefore, frequent voiding occurs.

- Bladder control and toilet training are not encouraged until sphincter control is achieved (usually after 2 years of age).

- Bladder capacity increases with age:
  Infants - 60 cc
  Toddlers - 285 - 400 cc
  Schoolage - 840 -1000 cc

- Disorders of the GU system cause fluid and electrolyte imbalances, inefficient clearance of medications, and build up of waste products in the body. Treatment and correction of disorders must occur promptly if long-term complications and possibly death are to be prevented.

II. Specific Genitourinary Disorders

Congenital Genitalia Defects

    a. **Description** - The malformation and poor differentiation of external and/or internal sex organs.

    b. **Signs and Symptoms** - Ambiguous genitalia; may be classified as masculinized female, incompletely masculinized male, true hermaphrodite, and mixed dysgenesis

    c. **Diagnostic Procedures** - Diagnosed by buccal smear, chromosomalanalysis, gonadal biopsy to determine sex, surgical observation of internal organs (laparotomy)

    d. **Medical Interventions**

      – **Medications** - Administer appropriate sex hormones to assist with development of secondary sex characteristics.

      – **Treatments** - Psychological support

      – **Surgery** - May include reconstruction of vagina or penis; gender assignment (usually female) prior to testosterone surge that occurs on postdelivery day 12

    e. **Nursing Interventions**

      – **Assessment and Actions**

        • Be alert to signs and symptoms.

        • Assess vital signs, I & O, postoperatively

        • Provide a method for reducing discomfort.

      – **Teaching**

        • Explain diagnosis to parents and long-term implications.

        • Explain surgical reconstruction and timing.

        • Teach parents about medication prescribed (drug, dose, route, time, and side effects).

      – **Emotional Care**

        • Provide parents with time for grieving.

        • Promote bonding between infant and parents.

        • Promote child's self-esteem and body image, age appropriate.

        • Provide support to family and child.

        • Provide support group information to family.

    f. **Potential Complications** - Emotional stress for parents and child, malignant degeneration of organs

2. CRYPTORCHIDISM

    a. **Description** - The failure of one or both testes to descend into the scrotal sac. The teste may be delayed in descending and return without treatment or actually be absent or irretractable. It is very common in pre-term males.

    b. **Signs and Symptoms** - Empty scrotal sac on palpation

   c. **Diagnostic Procedures** - Diagnosed through repeated manual examination of scrotal contents over the first two years of life; most testes typically descend by the age of one

   d. **Medical Interventions**
      - **Medications** - Administer antibiotics postoperatively.
      - **Treatments** - Unnecessary
      - **Surgery** - Surgical replacement (orchioplexy) before 3 years of age to preserve testes production of sperm

   e. **Nursing Interventions**
      - **Assessment and Actions**
         • Assess newborn and male children less than one year of age for scrotal content.
         • Postoperatively monitor vital signs, hydration, level of comfort (use bed cradle to prevent pressure on surgical area), observe for signs of infection.
         • Provide method for reducing discomfort.
      - **Teaching**
         • Discuss abnormality with parents and treatment regimen.
      - **Emotional Care**
         • Discuss infertility of child with parents if appropriate.
         • Provide support to family and child.

   f. **Potential Complications -** Infertility, long-term increased potential for neoplastic changes if teste(s) are not replaced in sac or removed

3. HYPOSPADIAS/EPISPADIAS

   a. **Description** - The malformation of the external urethral opening of the penis. The defect may be along the ventral surface (hypospadias) or along the dorsal surface (epispadias) and may be a small or severe defect.

   b. **Signs and Symptoms -** Abnormal location of urethral opening of penis on inspection

   c. **Diagnostic Procedures -** Diagnosis by inspection

   d. **Medical Interventions**
      - **Medications** - Administer antibiotics postoperatively
      - **Treatments** - Unnecessary
      - **Surgery** - Perform surgical repair of urethral opening between 6 and 18 months of age.

   e. **Nursing Interventions**
      - **Assessment and Actions**
         • Assess newborn male for any abnormality of urethral opening.
         • Postoperatively monitor vital signs, hydration status, signs of infection; prevent tension or pulling of catheter, monitor urine output

- Provide method for reducing pain.
- Assess for signs indicating potential pain.
- **Teaching**
  - Explain abnormality to parents and discuss treatment regimen.
- **Emotional Care**
  - Provide support to family and child.

f. **Potential Complications** - Scarring, fistulas, abnormality in physical appearance and function

Acquired Disorders

1. ACUTE GLOMERULONEPHRITIS

a. **Description** - An inflammation of the renal glomeruli believed to be related to an autoimmune complex disease. It typically follows a Group A Beta hemolytic streptococcal infection (usually upper respiratory or skin). It is more commonly seen in children from 4-7 years of age.

b. **Signs and Symptoms** - Symptoms appear approximately 10 days after streptococcal skin or respiratory infection and include periorbital edema, hypertension, anorexia, coke-colored and cloudy urine, irritability, headaches, proteinuria, hematuria; if disease progresses may develop oliguria, and generalized edema (anasarca)

c. **Diagnostic Procedures** - Diagnosed by urinalysis which reveals red cell casts, protein, elevated BUN and creatinine; blood studies reveal positive ASLO titer and hemoconcentration

d. **Medical Interventions**
   - **Medications** - Administer antihypertensives and antibiotics as needed.
   - **Treatments** - Prevent complications of renal disease, promote bedrest, may restrict dietary sodium; may require peritoneal dialysis
   - **Surgery** - Unnecessary

e. **Nursing Interventions**
   - **Assessment and Actions**
     - Be alert to signs and symptoms.
     - Implement bedrest, nutritional monitoring, and prevention of secondary infection.
     - Monitor vital signs, fluid and electrolytes, and weigh every day.
     - Assess for signs of CNS involvement (headaches, dizziness, seizures), note urinary output and color.
     - Provide skin care to prevent breakdown.
     - Administer medications as ordered.

- Assess for signs indicating potential complications (change in urine output abnormal cardiac or respiratory sounds, change in neurostates).

  - **Teaching**
    - Explain diagnosis to parents and child and allow time for questions.
    - Explain normal progression of disease to parents and child: edematous stage followed by diuretic stage, and then, return to wellness.
    - Teach parents importance of complying with diet therapy and what foods and/or fluids are restricted.
    - Discuss with parents importance of follow-up visits.
    - Teach parents about medications prescribed (drug, dose, route, time, and side effects).

  - **Emotional Care**
    - Provide support to family and child.

  f. **Potential Complications** - During acute phase (the first 4-10 days) may cause skin breakdown, encephalopathy, cardiac enlargement, pulmonary edema, and acute renal failure; may develop chronic renal disease

2. **ENURESIS**

   a. **Description** - Involuntary urination in a child who is at the age to achieve bladder control (primary enuresis) or has achieved bladder control (secondary enuresis). It may occur at night during sleep (nocturnal enuresis) and may be due to organic or nonorganic factors (disease process, infection, familial tendency, or stress). It is more frequently seen in boys. Diurnal enuresis in children over the age of five years is usually associated with an organic problem.

   b. **Signs and Symptoms -** Voiding involuntarily after the age of 4-5 years

   c. **Diagnostic Procedures** - Diagnosed by determining cause; may perform the following tests: urinalysis, urine C&S, x-ray to rule out mass or obstruction, psychological review

   d. **Medical Interventions**
      - **Medications** - May administer imipramine, DDAVP, or use antibiotics (if UTI is the cause)
      - **Treatments** - Treat according to cause; may include conditioning techniques (alarm mattress), bladder training exercises, psychotherapy.
      - **Surgery** - Surgical repair performed if due to obstruction or malformation in urinary tract.

   e. **Nursing Interventions**
      - **Assessment and Actions**
        - Be alert for signs and symptoms.

- Assess for signs of child abuse or sexual abuse.
- Assist with identifying cause by obtaining thorough bladder history (age of toilet training and method, infections, frequency of voiding).
- Assess for signs indicating potential complications.
  - **Teaching**
    - Explain diagnosis and treatment regimen to parents.
    - Encourage limiting fluids prior to bedtime, setting up a schedule for toileting, and teach bladder training exercises.
    - Teach parents about medication prescribed (drug, dose, route, time, and side effects).
  - **Emotional Care**
    - Identify and discuss parents' and child's feelings about problem.
    - Assist in identifying stressors in child's life and offer ways to reduce stress.
    - Promote child's self esteem and diminish guilty feelings.
    - Provide support to family and child.

  f. **Potential Complications**- Emotional stress, poor sense of self esteem, social isolation, urinary tract infections if obstruction is the cause

3. NEPHROTIC SYNDROME

  a. **Description** - Damage to the glomerular structure of the kidneys causing proteinuria, hypoalbuminemia, hyperlipidemia and edema. It usually follows a previous infection. It may be classified according to duration and kidney damage (minimal change nephrotic syndrome, secondary nephrotic syndrome, or congenital nephrotic syndrome). It is more commonly seen in children 2 - 3 years of age. The prognosis is good but the child may experience a relapse.

  b. **Sign and Symptoms -** Edema of face, abdomen, extremities; increase in weight, perineal edema, diarrhea, scanty dark-colored urine, lethargy, fatigue, hematuria, azotemia, proteinuria, hypovolemia; may experience respiratory difficulty if ascites is extreme

  c. **Diagnostic Procedures -** Diagnosed by presence of proteinuria, hematuria, elevated BUN, decreased creatinine clearances, renal biopsy reveals disease process

  d. **Medical Interventions**
    - **Medications** - Administer antibiotics specific to organism; long-term corticosteroid therapy, immunosuppressant therapy, diuretics, and cytoxan pulses (small doses of cytoxan given quickly with hydration pre- and post-administration) may be utilized.

- **Treatments** - Hospitalization may be necessary initially, promote rest, provide diet with minimal salt.
- **Surgery** - Unnecessary unless renal biopsy (punch or wedge resection) is indicated

e. Nursing Interventions
- **Assessment and Actions**
  - Be alert to signs and symptoms.
  - While hospitalized maintain bedrest , skin integrity, hydration status, monitor vital signs and weight, promote nutrition, monitor electrolyte levels, elevate edematous areas above level of heart.
  - Administer medications as ordered.
  - Maintain diet as ordered.
  - Anticipate diuretic phase within 1-3 weeks after symptoms appear.
  - Assess for signs indicating potential complications.
- **Teaching**
  - Explain diagnosis and discuss treatment regimen to family.
  - Emphasize importance of bedrest, good skin care and treatment regimen while at home.
  - Instruct parents on home monitoring of urine for albumin.
  - Teach parent about signs indicating potential complications.
- **Emotional Care**
  - Foster normal development of child.
  - Provide support to family and child.

f. Potential Complications - Relapse, infections, skin breakdown, social isolation (if frequent relapses occur), chronic renal disease, shock (from electrolyte imbalance), death if untreated

4. URINARY TRACT INFECTION (UTI)

a. **Description** - An infection of the urinary tract (urethra, ureters, bladder, kidneys). It may be acute, chronic, recurrent, or develop into a more severe GU disorder if left undetected or untreated. Kidney involvement often results from an ascending infection. It occurs more frequently in females due to the shorter urethra.

b. **Signs and Symptoms -** May be asymptomatic, particularly in chronic form; symptoms often age-dependent: *infants* - vomiting, diarrhea, FTT (Failure to Thrive), febrile episode, change in voiding habit and odor; *children* - dysuria, incontinence, increased frequency, enuresis, vomiting, fever, cloudy and strong smelling urine, flank pain, urgency

c. **Diagnostic Procedures -** Diagnosed by positive urine culture and sensitivity (C&S) and x-ray (if obstruction or defect is present)

   d. **Medical Interventions**
      - **Medications** - Administer antibiotic therapy (sulfonamide, ampicillin, amoxicillin).
      - **Treatments** - Increase fluid intake, monitor I&O.
      - **Surgery** - Surgical correction of defect or obstruction is performed if present.

   e. **Nursing Interventions**
      - **Assessment and Actions**
        • Be alert to signs and symptoms.
        • Assess for signs of sexual abuse.
        • Obtain thorough history to assist in determining causative factor.
        • Assess for signs indicating potential complications (altered urine output color or frequency).
      - **Teaching**
        • Explain diagnosis and discuss treatment regimen with parents and child.
        • Teach parents about medications prescribed (drug, dose, route, time, and side effects) and importance of administering antibiotics for 10 days, or the time prescribed.
        • Teach parents to monitor for signs of recurrence and to promote rest.
        • Teach parents to avoid using bubble bath and harsh detergents.
        • Teach female patients to wipe from front to back to avoid contamination from stool organisms.
        • Teach sexually-active females to urinate before and after intercourse.
      - **Emotional Care**
        • Provide support to family and child.

   f. **Potential Complications** - May lead to renal disease and renal failure if it is recurrent or becomes chronic.

5. **VESICOURETERAL REFLUX**

   a. **Description** - The back flow of urine from the bladder into the ureters and often into the kidneys. It can be due to a congenital malformation, obstruction, infection, or neurologic dysfunction. It may be graded according to area of reflux (Grade 1-5).

   b. **Signs and Symptoms** - Same as for UTI

   c. **Diagnostic Procedures** - Intravenous pyelogram reveals defect, voiding cystourethrogram and/or cystoscopy allows for visualization of defect.

  d. **Medical Interventions**
    — **Medications** - Administer antibiotics to prevent/treat infection.
    — **Treatments** - Teach bladder emptying exercise.
    — **Surgery** - May require surgical correction of defect or obstruction.

  e. **Nursing intervention**
    — **Assessment and Actions**
      • Be alert to signs and symptoms.
      • Postoperatively monitor vital signs, I&O, comfort level, and for signs of infection.
      • Assess for signs indicating potential complications.
    — **Teaching**
      • Explain diagnosis to parents and child and discuss treatment regimen.
      • Teach parents about medication prescribe (drug, dose, route, time, and side effects) and importance of maintaining compliance.
      • Instruct parents on watching for the recurring UTI, encouraging child to increase fluid intake, establishing a voiding schedule, and completely emptying bladder.
    — **Emotional Care**
      • Provide support to parents and child.

  f. **Potential Complications** - Renal disease

7

ENDOCRINE DISORDERS

I. General Concepts

- The endocrine system is composed of chemical secretions (hormones) manufactured by specific cells in the body and target cells which receive the secretions through different modes of transport and respond accordingly.

- It functions to regulate metabolism, growth, reproduction and sexual development, as well as, allows the body to maintain fluid and electrolyte balances and respond to stress.

- Endocrine glands include adrenal glands, ovaries, pancreas, parathyroid gland, pituitary gland, testes, and thyroid gland.

- Hormone secretion is based on a negative feedback loop throughout the body.

- The endocrine system plays a vital role in the child's growth and development.

- Disorders of the endocrine system may be due to a variety of factors and may be congenital or acquired; acute or chronic.

- Disorders may cause hyper- or hyposecretion of hormones.

- Early detection and treatment of disorders can limit many of the long-term effects.

- Discharge planning is vital to provide in order to assist the family and child with coping, compliance and appropriate home management.

II. Specific Endocrine Disorders

Acquired Disorders

1. DIABETES MELLITUS

   a. Description - The inability of the pancreas to secrete sufficient amounts of insulin. It may be due to genetic abnormality, autoimmune disorder, illness or stress. Type I Diabetes (IDDM - Insulin Dependent Diabetes Mellitus) is more common in children and young adults.

   b. Signs and Symptoms - Polyuria, polyphagia, polydipsia, hyperglycemia, glycosuria (with or without ketonuria), weight loss, fatigue, irritability, enuresis

   c. Diagnostic Procedures - Diagnosed by detecting glycosuria, fasting blood glucose less than 120 mg/dL, normal or elevated serum insulin levels, elevated hemoglobin A_1c

d. Medical Interventions

   – **Medications** - Administration of insulin; may require IV fluid resuscitation if in ketoacidosis

   – **Treatments** - Monitor blood and urine for glucose, protein and ketones; maintain diet following exchange list; encourage daily exercise regimen.

   – **Surgery** - Unnecessary

e. Nursing Interventions

   – **Assessment and Actions**

   - Be alert to signs and symptoms.
   - Monitor vital signs, blood and urine glucose, hydration status, level of consciousness, change in moods.
   - Encourage participation by child in controlling illness:
     - Preschoolers should be able to help with cleansing site for injection.
     - Schoolage children should be able to draw up and administer own insulin and monitor urine and blood with guidance.
     - Adolescents should be able to select food and make decisions regarding insulin needs during illness, exercise, and stress.
   - Discuss importance of compliance to treatment regimen, (problems tend to arise, especially in adolescence).
   - Assess for signs indicating potential complications.

- **Teaching**
  - Provide family and child with information about diagnosis and treatment regimen.
  - Prepare family and child for discharge by teaching:
    - Administration of insulin including type, amount, frequency, administration of injection, injection sites
    - Urine and blood monitoring and charting of these records
    - Meal planning and how to use the exchange list
    - How stress, illness, exercise, and growth affect insulin needs
    - Signs of imbalance and how to treat
      - **Hypoglycemia** - Rapid onset of symptoms, serum glucose less than 60 mg/dL, shakiness, irritability, dizziness, sweating, headache, tachycardia, shallow respirations, hunger, paleness, may lead to coma and death. **Treatment** - administer simple sugar immediately (orange juice, sugar, honey, candy, Coke); if insulin reaction occurs, administer glucagon
      - **Hyperglycemia** - Gradual onset of symptoms, serum glucose less than 250 mg/d, weakness, drowsiness, lethargy, nausea, thirst, Kussmaul respirations, fruity breath, confusion, polyuria, dry skin and mucous membranes, weak and thready pulse, may lead to acidosis, coma and death. **Treatment** - administer regular insulin, increase fluids. If DKA is present, hospitalization may be necessary to return to fluid and electrolyte balance
    - Importance of exercise and foot care
    - Importance of avoiding injuries
- **Emotional Care**
  - Allow time for questions and concerns about diagnosis.
  - Encourage parent to allow child as much independence as possible in treatment regime.
  - Promote self care.
  - Promote normal growth and development.
  - Discuss with family and child concerns about disease process.
  - Provide support to family and child.
  - Provide support group information to family.

  f. **Potential Complications** - Neurological complications, vascular changes and poor wound healing, retinal and kidney damage, impotence, death

2. HYPOPITUITARISM (GROWTH HORMONE HYPOSECRETION)

a. **Description** - A decrease in hormonal secretions from the pituitary gland. It is most commonly associated with a previous insult to the pituitary area (tumor, infection, radiation treatment).

b. **Signs and Symptoms** - Retarded linear growth with normal weight for age after first year of life; retaining youthful appearance; delay in appearance of permanent teeth, delayed sexual development, premature aging; if tumor-related -- may exhibit signs of headache or visual disturbances

c. **Diagnostic Procedures** - Diagnosed by assessing the family history for short stature, reviewing history of child's birth, reviewing child's growth (height and weight) from infancy, reviewing skeletal and skull x-ray to assess bone ossification and presence of masses; CT scan may be used to localize tumor or lesion; endocrine studies reveal decreased or absent growth hormone

d. **Medical Interventions**
   - **Medications** - Administration of biosynthetic growth hormones as soon as detected
   - **Treatments** - Monitor response to medication
   - **Surgery** - Surgical removal or irradiation of tumor, if indicated

e. **Nursing Interventions**
   - **Assessment and Actions**
     • Assist with detection by plotting growth chart and sexual development.
     • Continue to monitor growth once treatment is implemented.
     • Assess for signs indicating potential complications.
   - **Teaching**
     • Discuss diagnostic tests that may be required.
     • Discuss diagnosis and long-term treatment regimen with child and family.
     • Discuss need for frequent injections (usually 3 times per week) with child and family.
     • Discuss signs and symptoms of hypoglycemia and treatment.
     • Inform that most children who are treated will eventually reach an adult height but puberty is often delayed by 1-2 years.
   - **Emotional Care**
     • Encourage family to treat child at appropriate level for age even though they appear smaller.
     • Promote positive self esteem in child (especially adolescent age group).
     • Provide support to family and child.

f. **Potential Complications** - Social isolation, emotional problems, delayed growth; if untreated, child will never attain normal size

3. HYPOTHYROIDISM

a. Description - An abnormally low production of hormones from the thyroid gland. It may be congenital or acquired, acute or chronic. It affects 1 in 4 newborns and is often referred to as cretinism.

b. Signs and Symptoms - Newborn asymptomatic initially, if untreated: slow growth, irregular movements, brittle hair, dry, flaky skin, small forehead with eyes widely spread (infancy), cold skin, bradycardia, sleepiness, fatigue, constipation, nonpitting myxedema, large tongue, hoarse voice, may lead to mental retardation if undetected and untreated

c. Diagnostic Procedures - Diagnosed by finding decreased T_4 (thyroxine), elevated TSH levels, delayed epiphyseal development, decreased creatinine clearance; may use radioisotope of iodine to detect thyroid function

d. Medical Interventions
  - **Medications** - Administration of thyroid hormone (Levothyroxine).
  - **Treatments** - Monitor response to medication therapy.
  - **Surgery** - Unnecessary

e. Nursing Interventions
  - **Assessment and Actions**
    - Be alert to signs and symptoms.
    - Refer parents for genetic counseling.
    - Assess for signs indicating potential complications.
    - Maintain accurate growth charts.
    - Monitor for achievement of developmental milestones.
  - **Teaching**
    - Provide information to parents and child regarding disorder, treatment regimen and effects on child.
    - Teach parents about medication prescribed (drug, dose, route, time, and side effects), need for compliance, and possible signs of overdose.
    - Inform that child may appear "hyperactive" when compared to previous activity level
  - **Emotional Care**
    - Provide support to family and child.

f. Potential Complications - If untreated: growth retardation, developmental delays, irreversible mental retardation

4. HYPERTHYROIDISM

a. Description - The oversecretion of thyroid hormone. It has an unknown etiology. It is more common in adolescence.

b. **Signs and Symptoms** - Gradual onset of symptoms: increased hunger, weight loss, constant movement, nervousness, goiter (in some cases), sleeplessness, tachycardia, cardiomegaly, vomiting, diarrhea, warm and moist skin, intolerance to heat, exophthalmos, staring expression, weakness

c. **Diagnostic Procedures** - Diagnosed by presence of increased T_4 and T_3 levels, decreased TSH levels, mass may be palpable on thyroid gland, enlargement of gland on CT, increased uptake of ^{131}I (radioactive iodine isotope)

d. **Medical Interventions**
   - **Medications** - Administration of antithyroid medication (propyl-thiouracil), propranolol, iodide
   - **Treatments** - Maintain diet with increased calories, carbohydrates and vitamins; radiation therapy may be necessary.
   - **Surgery** - Surgical removal of thyroid (thyroidectomy) may be necessary

e. **Nursing Interventions**
   - **Assessment and Actions**
     - Be alert to signs and symptoms.
     - Observe for signs of thyrotoxicosis (thyroid storm): sudden vomiting, irritability, tachycardia, hypertension, and elevated temperature.
   - **Teaching**
     - Explain diagnosis and treatment regimen to parents and child.
     - Assist parents with providing for increased nutritional needs, and understanding problems of hyperthermia and possible behavior problems.
     - Teach parents about medications prescribed (drug, dose, route, time, and side effects).
   - **Emotional Care**
     - Provide support to family and child.

f. **Potential Complications** - Thyroidtoxicosis - thyroid crisis; signs and symptoms: restlessness, vomiting, diarrhea, tachycardia, hypertension, hyperthermia, may lead to coma and death if untreated; usually due to an illness or discontinuing antithyroid medication. **Treatment:** Administration of antithyroid medication and propranolol

Congenital Disorder

1. PHENYLKETONURIA (PKU)

a. **Description** - A genetic error of metabolism that occurs in 1 in 15,000 births. It is carried by an autosomal recessive gene and 1 in 50-100 people carry the gene. These children have absence of phenylalanine hydroxylase (a hepatic enzyme) which allows the conversion of phenylalanine to tyrosine. Abnormal byproducts accumulate in the bloodstream and are excreted via urine and sweat. They may also accumulate in the CSF or body tissue. The level rises with protein ingestion and leads to neural damage and mental retardation.

b. **Signs and Symptoms** - Undiagnosed infants present moderate to severe mental retardation due to degeneration of the brain and demyelinization of the nerves. Urine has a musty odor; may have eczema or seborrhea, seizures, hyperactivity, bizarre personality, and behavior problems. Child is usually blonde, blue-eyed, and fair-skinned due to failure to produce melanin.

c. **Diagnostic Procedures** - Newborn screening is the most effective method. Phenylalanine levels 16-20 mg/d, a serum tyrosine level 3 mg/d, and phenylpyruvic acid and o-hydroxyphenylacetic acid in the urine are confirmation. Initial newborn screen may produce a false negative, rescreening at 14-28 days may be suggested. Questionable results should be referred for phenylalanine challenge.

d. **Medical Interventions**
   – **Medications** - None
   – **Treatments** - Dietary treatment is used for control; diet consists of amino acid restricted diet at least until brain growth is complete (7-8 years). Infants are given a reduced phenylalanine formula (Lofenlac®).
   – **Surgery** - Unnecessary

e. **Nursing Interventions**
   – **Assessment and Actions**
     • Be alert to signs and symptoms of PKU.
     • Assess nutritional, growth and developmental status.
     • Work closely with multidisciplinary team following child to ensure communication.
   – **Teaching**
     • Explain meaning of diagnosis and planned medical treatment plan including dietary restrictions.
   – **Emotional Care**
     • Encourage parents to have genetic counseling.
     • Provide support to child and family.

f. **Potential Complications** - Mental retardation, hyperactivity and other behavioral problems, altered growth, failure to achieve developmental milestones/tasks

8

MUSCULOSKELETAL DISORDERS

I. General Concepts

- The musculoskeletal system is made up of bones, joints, and muscles.

- It functions to provide movement, heat production, posture, support, protection, mineral storage, and production of blood.

- Muscle and skeletal tissue increase in size and density as the child ages.

- The skeletal system continues to grow and develop until after puberty is completed, and the epiphysis of long bones closes.

- The skeletal system heals more quickly in children than in adults.

- The musculoskeletal system is affected by nutritional intake and by other disease processes; for example, parathyroid disorders, renal disease, malabsorption syndrome.

II. Specific Treatments and Nursing Interventions

Cast

Utilized to immobilize extremity and promote alignment healing

- May be made of plaster or synthetic materials such as fiberglass.

- Prepare child for procedure, and describe sensations that may be felt (cold, wet, heavy).

- Assist with comfort measures and with resetting extremity.

- Provide warmth until cast is dried.

- Handle wet cast with palms of hands to prevent indentations.

- Elevate cast on pillows.

- Assess cast for odor, drainage, pain, and maintain smooth edges. Use petals if needed.

- Discourage the sticking of objects into cast to scratch extremity.

- Assess neurovascular status distal to cast (capilary refill, sensation, temperature, pulse, color).

- Discuss with child and family the limitations of wearing a cast.

- Teach crutch walking or means of mobilization.

- Promote safety while cast is in place.

- Discuss length of time cast will be in place.

- Before procedure, prepare child before removal of the cast and the appearance of extremity underneath the cast.

- If spica cast is utilized, never move child by picking up by bar; promote safety, identify method of transportation/mobilization for child, keep perineum clean, maintain hydration and increase fiber in diet to prevent constipation.

Fixation

Surgical placement of pins or wires to restore alignment and give support to extremity or affected bone

- May be internal or external pin placement.

- Internal placement requires monitoring for signs of infection and providing comfort measures.

- External placement requires pin site assessment and care and monitoring for discomfort and infection.

- Describe procedure to parent and child and what area will look like after placement.

- Discuss care of pins (as appropriate) and limitations fixation presents.

- Identify a method of mobilization for child and teach crutch walking.

- Provide safety measures for child.

- Discuss length of time fixation will need to be utilized.

Traction

Utilization of weights and pulleys, straps or pins to return bone or muscle to normal position; includes manual traction, skin traction and skeletal traction

- Prepare child and family for type of traction utilized.
- Describe limitations traction presents (immobilization).
- Discuss length of time traction will be needed.
- Promote normal growth and development for child and enhance socialization when possible.
- Monitor skin for signs of infection or ulcerations.
- Assess circulation and neurological status to distal extremity.
- Maintain proper body alignment and position in bed.
- Maintain free hanging weights.
- Promote comfort, nutrition and hydration (prevents constipation).
- Teach child how to use trapeze correctly.
- Place nurse call light within reach.
- Provide safe environment (side rails up).

III. Specific Musculoskeletal Disorders

Congenital Disorders

1. CLUBFOOT (TALIPES)

a. **Description** - A unilateral or bilateral congenital malposition of the foot or ankle.

b. **Signs and Symptoms** - Visual detection of incorrect positioning of the foot or ankle; foot or ankle cannot be manually positioned into normal alignment and is rigid to movement

c. **Diagnostic Procedures** - Diagnosed by characteristic physical findings and inability to manually return foot/ankle into alignment

d. **Medical Interventions**

- **Medications** - Administer antibiotics postoperatively.
- **Treatments** - Return foot to functioning position as soon as detected; mild forms may require daily ROM, massage, and placement of corrective shoes (Denis-Browne splints), some forms may require serial casting, corrective strapping.
- **Surgery** - More severe forms may require surgical correction.

e. **Nursing Interventions** - *(See previous section referring to casts)*

- **Assessment and Actions**
  - Be alert to signs and symptoms indicating disorder.

- Assess child postoperatively for discomfort and provide method for reducing discomfort.
- Postoperatively, monitor vital signs and neurological, circulatory status of distal area.
- Assess for signs indicating potential complications.

    – **Teaching**
- Explain diagnosis and treatment regimen to family.
- Instruct family on care of the child: ROM, proper placement and care of the child in Denis-Browne splints (limitations of movement, care in turning or carrying, time of application).
- If casting or strapping is required, instruct parents on care of casts/straps and affected area, frequency in which cast/straps will be changed, and signs or symptoms which require further medical assessment.
- If surgical correction is required prepare child and parents for what to expect.
- Prepare family for discharge and necessary home care of child with a cast.

    – **Emotional Care**
- Provide support to family and child.

   f. **Potential Complications** - Infection, foot deformity and scarring

2. CONGENITAL HIP DYSPLASIA

   a. **Description** - The congenital displacement of the femoral head from the acetabulum. It may be categorized as: preluxation, subluxation, or dislocation. It is more commonly seen in females than in males. It may be a unilateral or bilateral defect.

   b. **Signs and Symptoms** - Unequal gluteal or thigh folds, discrepancy in leg length, diminished ability to abduct affected side, pain with diapering, positive click or popping with Ortolani and Barlow test; if undetected in infancy, may note leg length discrepancy in ambulating child as well as uneven gait (Trendelenberg gait)

   c. **Diagnostic Procedures** - Diagnosed by characteristic physical assessment findings and x-ray which shows defect

   d. **Medical Interventions**
- **Medications** - If surgically corrected, administer antibiotics postoperatively.
- **Treatments** - Maintain hip in flexion and abduction (Pavlik harness, Frejka pillow, or casting).
- **Surgery** - Surgical reduction and reconstruction may be necessary if not treated early in life.

   e. **Nursing Interventions** - (See previous section referring to casts)

    – **Assessment and Actions**
- Be alert to signs and symptoms indicating disorder.

- If surgical reduction required, postoperatively monitor vital signs, circulation to area, for signs of infection.
- Provide method for reducing discomfort.
- Assess for signs indicating potential complications.

- **Teaching**
  - Explain diagnosis and discuss treatment regimen with parents.
  - Instruct parents on treatment regimen; teach how to care for child in harness or pillow device, encourage keeping skin and device dry and clean, monitoring for skin breakdown, discuss how to handle and care for child.
  - Teach cast care and handling, if appropriate.
  - Postoperatively,or after casting, teach means for mobilization.

- **Emotional Care**
  - Promote normal growth and development.
  - Provide support to family and child

f. **Potential Complications** - If left untreated, may cause permanent change in femoral head or acetabulum, avascular necrosis; if surgical interventions necessary, may encounter infection

3. **DUCHENNE'S MUSCULAR DYSTROPHY (PSEUDOHYPERTROPHIC MUSCULAR DYSTROPHY)**

a. **Description** - A sex-linked, inherited condition that primarily affects males which involves a progressive muscle weakness and wasting. Symptoms usually appear by 2-6 years of age.

b. **Signs and Symptoms** - Progressive muscle weakness beginning in spine, shoulders and hips, clumsiness, developmental delay or difficulty in gross motor activities, difficulty getting up from floor (Gower's sign), frequent falls, waddling gait, muscle atrophy, enlarged calf muscles; may later exhibit lordosis; muscle-wasting eventually affects all muscles of the body (including heart and respiratory system) death usually occurs by age 20 from heart failure or respiratory infection

c. **Diagnostic Procedures** - Diagnosed by detecting EMG myopathy, muscle biopsy reveals degeneration and variation in muscle size and increased amounts of connective tissue, serum enzyme tests reveal elevated CPK

d. **Medical Interventions**
  - **Medications** - Administer antibiotics to treat respiratory infections.
  - **Treatments** - Prevent complications and maintain child at optimal functioning level, utilize PT, promote diet therapy.
  - **Surgery** - May be required to release contractures.

e. **Nursing Interventions**
   - **Assessment and Actions**
     • Be alert to signs and symptoms.
     • Prepare child and parents for diagnostic testing.
     • Encourage exercise (swimming is excellent) and promote rest periods.
     • As disease progresses, provide care for patient on complete bedrest (skin care, ROM, pulmonary care).
     • Refer parents to genetic counseling.
     • Assess for signs indicating potential complications.
   - **Teaching**
     • Explain diagnosis and discuss treatment regimen with parents and child.
     • Explain progression of disease.
     • Teach child how to utilize and develop accessory breathing muscles (diaphragmatic breathing exercises) and utilize CPT as ordered.
     • Teach parents and child ROM exercises, application of braces and positioning to prevent contractures.
     • Teach parents to keep environment safe.
     • Teach parents and child how to use wheelchair.
   - **Emotional Care**
     • Assist parents with promoting child's independence.
     • Promote growth and development, self-care, and socialization as much as possible.
     • Provide support to family and child.
     • Provide support group information to family.
   f. **Potential Complications** - Contractures, obesity, infections, atrophy

4. **OSTEOGENESIS IMPERFECTA**
   a. **Description** - An autosomal dominant (more frequent) or autosomal recessive disorder in which there is a defect in the connective tissues and bone causing disorganized bone structure and, therefore, brittle or fragile bones. It ranges in severity of bone fragility.

   b. **Signs and Symptoms** - Depends upon severity and classification: frequent fractures, blue sclera, dentinogenesis, short stature, often exhibit several fractures or healed fractures on x-ray, may have hearing loss

   c. **Diagnostic Procedures** - Diagnosed by characteristic physical findings, reduced cortical thickness of shafts of long bones; elevated serum phrophosphate levels, and decreased platelet aggregation; often must rule out physical abuse due to multiple fractures noted on x-ray

   d. **Medical Interventions**
- **Medication** - Unnecessary
- **Treatments** - Prevent complications and treat fractures.
- **Surgery** - May require pinning of fractures (intramedullary rods) to strengthen area and permit correct alignment

   e. **Nursing Interventions**
- **Assessment and Actions**
  - Assess child's level of comfort and provide method for reducing discomfort
  - Assess child's ROM.
  - Assess limitations in ADLs.
  - Provide safe environment for child during hospitalization.
  - Refer parents for genetic counseling.
  - Assess for signs indicating potential complications.
- **Teaching**
  - Discuss diagnosis with family and child.
  - Discuss necessity for child's safety and importance of limiting contact sports.
  - Discuss chronicity of disease and how child may become somewhat less fragile with age.
  - Instruct child and family on how to apply and adapt to corrective devices that may be utilized: casts, braces, splints, hearing aids, glasses.
  - Encourage gentle care of child during ADLs.
  - Teach parent and child use of wheelchair as needed.
  - Discourage immobility to decrease atrophy and likelihood of refracture.
- **Emotional Care**
  - Promote growth and development.
  - Provide support to family and child.
  - Provide support group information to family.

   f. **Potential Complications** - Maligned bone healing causing deformity, hearing and/or vision loss, often confined to wheelchair as an adult; death if severe form of disease is acquired at birth

Acquired Disorders

1. FRACTURES

   a. **Description** - A break in the bone. It may be classified according to tissue injury and includes simple or closed, compound, or comminuted. The fractures that occur commonly in children include bends, buckles, complete, and greenstick fractures. If the epiphyseal plate is injured, bone growth may be affected.

b. **Signs and Symptoms** - Pain, swelling, decreased movement, numbness, tingling, deformity, ecchymosis

c. **Diagnostic Procedures** - Diagnosed by physical findings and x-ray which reveals abnormality in bone; lab values may reveal elevated serum bilirubin, decreased hemoglobin and hematocrit, may have elevated creatine alkaline phosphate, SGOT, and LDH, and elevated WBC

d. **Medical Interventions**

  – **Medications** - Administer antibiotics to minimize infection.

  – **Treatments** - Realign and immobilize (casting or traction) injured area.

  – **Surgery** - Surgical correction may be necessary (open reduction) with or without pinning.

e. **Nursing Interventions** - (See previous section referring to casts, traction and fixation)

  – **Assessment and Actions**

    • Be alert to signs and symptoms indicating disorder.

    • Provide method for reducing discomfort.

    • Monitor for signs of infection.

    • Assist with identifying how child will ambulate if leg is involved.

    • Assess distal area for neurovascular functioning.

    • Assess for signs indicating potential complications.

  – **Teaching**

    • Explain diagnosis and discuss treatment regimen with parents and child.

    • Prepare child for casting procedure and discuss length of time cast will be in place.

    • If traction is necessary, prepare child and family and instruct on immobilization (see previous section on Special Treatments).

    • Encourage diet high in protein and calcium.

  – **Emotional Care**

    • Promote growth and development.

    • Provide support to family and child.

f. **Potential Complications** - Fat embolism, infection, altered growth in extremity

2. **JUVENILE RHEUMATOID ARTHRITIS**

a. **Description** - An inflammatory condition of the joints and connective tissue. It is chronic and usually occurs before puberty. It may involve one or more joints and cycles through remissions and exacerbations.

b. **Signs and Symptoms** - Nonmigratory swollen, tender joints that exhibit decrease in ROM (lasting 3 months or more); often the stiffness is worse in the morning (gelling); fever, erythematous rash, leukocytosis, iridocyclitis

c. Diagnostic Procedures - Diagnosed by characteristic physical findings and history of persistent symptoms for three months; x-ray reveals soft tissue swelling and regional osteoporosis; often necessary to rule out other disease processes (cancer, rheumatic fever, Lyme's disease)

d. Medical Interventions

- **Medications** - Administration of nonsteroidal anti-inflammatory drugs (NSAIDs), slower acting antirheumatic drugs, corticosteroids, cytotoxic medications, aspirin

- **Treatments** - Maintain ROM and comfort.

- **Surgery** - May require synovectomy, joint replacement or joint fusion

e. Nursing Interventions

- **Assessment and Actions**
  - Assess limitations in ROM.
  - Assess for activities that cause exacerbations.
  - Provide method for reducing discomfort.
  - Assess for signs indicating potential complications.

- **Teaching**
  - Discuss diagnosis and chronicity with parents and child.
  - Instruct parents on home therapy, ROM exercises (passive ROM after inflammatory period), splinting of affected extremities, application of heat.
  - Instruct on methods for reducing discomfort.
  - Encourage application of warm compresses or warm paraffin or whirlpool therapy to joints.
  - Teach parents about medication prescribed (drug, dose, route, time, and side effects).

- **Emotional Care**
  - Promote growth and development and self-esteem of child.
  - Provide support group information to family.

f. Potential Complications - Contractures, cataracts, loss of joint mobility

3. LEGG-CALVE-PERTHES DISEASE

a. Description - A self-limiting disease in which localized ischemia causes avascular necrosis of the femoral head. It results in degeneration of the femoral head and may affect the growth plate. It progresses through four states: avascular stage, revascularization stage, reparative stage, and regenerative stage. It is most commonly seen during 4-8 years of age. It is often referred to as Coxa Plana or osteochondritis deformans juveniles.

b. Signs and Symptoms - May initially exhibit a limp, complain of soreness and pain in the hip joint, and display guarding or limitation in ROM.

c. Diagnostic Procedures - Diagnosed by evidence of deterioration of the femoral head by x-ray

d. Medical Interventions
 - **Medications** - Unnecessary
 - **Treatments** - Focuses on preservation of the joint and extremity throughout course of disease (may require 2 years of treatment), maintaining joint in acetabulum, placement of casts or braces to hold joint in abduction and internal rotation
 - **Surgery** - Surgical repair or replacement of joint may be necessary if joint becomes damaged.

e. Nursing Interventions
 - **Assessment and Actions**
   • Assess level of discomfort.
   • Limit ROM of affected extremity.
   • Assess skin for areas of breakdown due to brace.
   • Provide method for reducing discomfort.
   • Assess for signs indicating complications.
 - **Teaching**
   • Discuss diagnosis with family and child and long-term treatment requirements.
   • Instruct parents and child on importance of bedrest and compliance with treatment regimen.
   • Instruct on proper brace application and discourage weight bearing on affected extremity.
   • Teach crutch walking or identify mode for movement.
   • If bedrest and traction are necessary discuss with parent and child (see previous section on Special Treatments).
   • Prepare parents and child for discharge and home care.
 - **Emotional Care**
   • Promote growth and development.
   • Provide support to family and child.

f. Potential Complications - Loss of ROM, growth disturbance in affected limb

4. OSTEOMYELITIS

a. Description - An infection of the bone tissue usually preceded by an infection or injury somewhere in the body. It usually affects the long bones and may be an acute or chronic disease.

   b. Signs and Symptoms - Pain in affected area accompanied by guarding, swelling, warmth over area, fever, irritability, diarrhea

   c. Diagnostic Procedures - Diagnosed by presence of a positive blood culture, an increased ESR, presence of leukocytosis, x-ray reveals localized swelling

   d. Medical Interventions

     – **Medications** - Long-term antibiotic therapy (organism specified)

     – **Treatments** - Maintain bedrest, splint affected extremity.

     – **Surgery** - Surgical drainage of area or aspiration of fluid may be required.

   e. Nursing Interventions

     – **Assessment and Actions**

       • Monitor VS, hydration status, and level of comfort.

       • Maintain patent IV and administer antibiotics as scheduled (may be treated at home).

       • After treatment progresses and bone is infection free, slowly introduce ROM to extremity.

       • Provide method for reducing discomfort.

       • Assess for signs indicating potential complications.

     – **Teaching**

       • Discuss diagnosis and necessity for long-term antibiotic therapy (4-6 weeks).

       • Discuss with child and parents limitations: bedrest, immobilization of extremity, avoidance of weight bearing or use of affected extremity

     – **Emotional Care**

       • Promote growth and development and socialization.

       • Provide support to family and child.

   f. Potential Complications - Spread of infection to other sites, injury to bone, permanent loss of bone structure, growth abnormality or extremity

5. SLIPPED FEMORAL CAPITAL EPIPHYSIS (EPIPHYSIOLYSIS)

   a. Description - The displacement of the femoral head from the neck of the femur. It is caused by a shift in the epiphyseal plate. It typically occurs during a growth spurt and is more frequently seen in obese adolescents. It may occur unilaterally or bilaterally and can be an acute or chronic disorder. It may or may not be preceded by a traumatic injury to the area.

   b. Signs and Symptoms - Intermittent or constant hip or groin pain, decreased internal rotation of hip, decreased ROM of hip, limping

   c. Diagnostic Procedures - Diagnosed by physical findings and by visualizing displacement of femoral head on x-ray

d. Medical Interventions

- **Medications** - Unnecessary
- **Treatments** - Protect the joint and growth plate, preventing contractures.
- **Surgery** - May require internal fixation with pins, skeletal traction, or osteotomy

e. Nursing Interventions

- **Assessment and Actions**
  - Be alert to signs and symptoms.
  - Provide method for reducing discomfort.
  - Assess for signs indicating potential complications.
- **Teaching**
  - Discuss diagnosis with parents and child.
  - Explain limitations of disorder: no weight bearing on extremity, bedrest and traction.
  - Teach child crutch walking and about traction (see previous section on Special Treatments).
- **Emotional Care**
  - Promote growth, development and self-esteem.
  - Provide support to family and child.

f. Potential Complications - Altered growth in affected extremity, chronic pain or limping, avascular necrosis of area

6. SCOLIOSIS

a. Description - The lateral curvature of the spine. It may be a structural (progressive disorder requiring mechanical or surgical correction) or a nonstructural (nonprogressive and voluntarily correctable, often due to poor posture) disorder.

b. Signs and Symptoms - Visual malalignment of the spine, sternum is not in midline, visible unilateral hump noted on posterior along spine when child bends forward, hips are not bilaterally even in height; often asymptomatic

c. Diagnostic Procedures - Diagnosed by physical findings and confirmed by visible malalignment on x-ray

d. Medical Interventions

- **Medications** - Administer antibiotic postoperatively
- **Treatments** - Treatment depends upon type of disorder: Nonstructural scoliosis--exercises to improve muscle strength and posture, utilization of external brace; structural scoliosis--exercises, brace, electrical stimulation
- **Surgery** - Structural scoliosis may require surgical correction (spinal fusion, Harrington, Dwyer, or Luque instrumentation)

e. Nursing Interventions

– Assessment and Actions

- Provide screening to all teenagers, especially females, during physical examinations.
- Prepare child for wearing brace; describe fitting, hygiene, and when it can be removed.
- If surgery required, prepare child for surgical procedure and what to expect postoperatively.
- Postoperatively monitor child's VS, neuro and circulatory status, comfort level, hydration, nutrition, urinary elimination, and skin for signs of breakdown or infection; turn child by log-rolling and keep positioned in alignment.
- Assess for signs indicating potential complications.

– Teaching

- Explain diagnosis to parent and child.
- Explain treatment regimen and importance of compliance.
- Teach child exercise regimen and obtain return demonstration.
- Postoperative discharge education should include instructing child not to sit for long periods of time, to refrain from bending (squat instead), and to participate in only low impact activities.
- Teach importance of safety for child in brace.
- Prepare child and family for discharge and home care, including how to perform physical therapy.

– Emotional Care

- Assist child in identifying clothing that will conceal brace.
- Discuss child's feelings of having to wear brace.
- Promote child's self-esteem and development.
- Provide support to family and child.
- Provide support group information to family.

f. Potential Complications - Permanent skeletal deformity

9

COMMUNICABLE DISEASES

I. General Concepts

- Communicable diseases are caused by those infectious agents which are passed or transmitted via animate or inanimate objects (reservoir) to a host and which cause illness of that host.

- Transmission may be through direct or indirect contact with infected item.

- Children are more susceptible to communicable diseases due to the immaturity in their immune system and their increased interaction with the environment.

- Communicable diseases can occur at any age.

- Communicable diseases require the nurse to attempt to prevent the occurrence, identify the disease quickly, provide treatment, prevent the spread , and prevent any possible complications.

- Many communicable diseases may also be prevented by improved handwashing, proper hygiene, and limited exposure to other children or objects the infected children have played with while in the contagious stage of the disease.

- Many communicable diseases can be prevented by immunizing the child.

II. Prevention of Communicable Diseases

Immunizations

1. The following immunization schedule should be adhered to:

RECOMMENDED SCHEDULE OF VACCINATIONS FOR ALL CHILDREN							
Vaccine		2 Months	4 Months	6 Months	12 Months	15 Months	4-6 Years (Before school entry)
DTP		DTP	DTP	DTP		DTP*	DTP
POLIO		POLIO	POLIO			POLIO*	POLIO
MMR						MMR†	MMR¶
HIB Option 1 § Option 2 §		HIB HIB	HIB HIB	HIB	HIB	HIB	
Vaccine	Birth	1-2 Months	4 Months	6-18 Months			
HB Option 1 Option 2	HB	HB‡ HB‡	HB‡	HB‡ HB‡			

DTP: Diphteria, Tetanus, and Pertussis Vaccine
Polio: Live Oral Polio Vaccine drops (OPV)
or Killed (Inactivated) Polio Vaccine shots (IPV)

MMR: Measles, Mumps, and Rubella Vaccine
HIB: Haemophilus b Conjugate Vaccine
HB: Hepatitis B Vaccine

* Many experts recommend these vaccines at 18 months.
† In some areas this dose of MMR vaccine may be given at 12 months.
¶ Many experts recommend this dose of MMR vaccine be given between entry to middle school or junior high school.
§ HIB vaccine is given in either a 4-dose schedule (1) or a 3-dose schedule (2), depending upon the type of vaccine used.
‡ Hepatitis B vaccine can be given simultaneously with DTP, Polio, MMR, and Haemophilus b Conjugate Vaccine at the same visit.

Source: U.S. Department of Health and Human Services, Public Health Services, Centers for Disease Control. (1991). What you need to know. Atlanta: Author.

2. Parents must sign a consent form prior to immunization administration.
3. Child should be screened prior to administration to ensure:
   a. Immunizations are up to date
   b. Child is not currently sick or does not have chronic illness
   c. Previous reactions not experienced
   d. No previous history of seizures or cranial anomalies. If there is a question about whether child should receive immunization, consult physician
4. Make parents aware of normal and abnormal side effects and when to seek further assistance for child if reaction occurs.

5. Children with depressed immune systems or who have a fever should not be given immunizations.
6. If immunization schedule is interrupted, continue with last immunization.

Immunity may be categorized as follows:

1. ARTIFICIALLY ACQUIRED IMMUNITY

Host is exposed to infectious organism artificially introduced into the host's body, host then builds antibodies against future organism contamination. Duration of immunity varies and booster immunizations may be required. Example: Childhood immunization

2. ARTIFICIALLY ACQUIRED PASSIVE IMMUNITY

Host is injected with antibodies to specific infectious agent, duration of immunity varies from weeks to months. Example: gamma globulin, hepatitis B immune globulin.

3. NATURALLY ACQUIRED ACTIVE IMMUNITY

Host is directly exposed to organism in external environment and builds antibodies after infected, duration of immunity lasts throughout life. Example: varicella zoster, parotitis

4. NATURALLY ACQUIRED PASSIVE IMMUNITY

Host is exposed to antibodies through placenta while still in utero or through breast milk, protection lasts first 3 - 4 months of life

III. Pediatric Communicable Diseases

A. Bacterial Infections

1. CORNYBACTERIUM DIPTHERIA (DIPTHERIA)

a. **Age Typically Affected** - Infants and young children who have not been immunized

b. **Signs and Symptoms** - Sore throat, visible membrane formation in nasopharynx area, may effect the nasal, tonsilar, pharyngeal, or laryngeal areas; malaise, anorexia, low-grade fever, lymphadenopathy, hoarseness, cough

c. **Communicable Period** - Variable, usually 2 - 4 weeks after symptoms appear

d. **Seasonal Incidence** - Common in fall and winter

e. **Transmission** - Direct contact by sneezing, coughing, and talking with infected person

f. **Nursing Interventions** - Strict isolation, medication therapy, complete bedrest, observe respiratory status, high carbohydrate diet, increased fluid intake

g. **Potential Complication** - Approximately 50% of children infected also develop myocardial complications, also may have temporary neuritis and soft palate paralysis

2. PERTUSSIS (WHOOPING COUGH)

   a. **Age Typically Affected** - Less common in immunized children, may affect infants and children up to 4 years old

   b. **Signs and Symptoms** - Upper respiratory infection signs and symptoms, low-grade fever, paroxysmal coughing worsens and is most frequent at night, often sounds like a whooping crane, child may become cyanotic during episode, mucous plug may be expelled during coughing episode, often followed by vomiting

   c. **Communicable Period -** One week prior and 3 - 4 weeks after symptoms appear

   d. **Seasonal Incidence** - Spring and summer

   e. **Transmission** - Droplets or contact with contaminated inanimate object

   f. **Nursing Interventions** - Isolate child, bedrest with quiet environment, humidified air, increase fluid intake, monitor airway, antimicrobial medication administration to decrease communicability

   g. **Potential Complications** - Pneumonia, malnutrition, seizures, rectal prolapse, may cause death if severe obstruction occurs

3. SCARLET FEVER (SCARLATINA)

   a. **Age Typically Affected** - Children 6 - 12 years

   b. **Signs and Symptoms** - Initially high fever, bright red macules that diminish with pressure, often concentrated in areas near folds (groin, axilla), enlarged tonsils covered by exudate, beefy red strawberry tongue, after 1 week skin begins to flake

   c. **Communicable Period** - Variable, greater during acute respiratory symptoms phase until initiation of antibiotic therapy

   d. **Seasonal Incidence** - Winter and early spring more common

   e. **Transmission** - Contact with infected person or respiratory secretions, may also contract through infected articles

   f. **Nursing Interventions** - Antibiotic administration, respiratory isolation, bedrest, oral hygiene, increase fluid intake, antipyretics administration prn.

   g. **Potential Complications** - Early detection and treatment may reduce these: cervical adenitis, otitis media, sinusitis, pneumonia, rheumatic fever, glomerulonephritis

4. TETANUS ("LOCKJAW")

   a. **Age Typically Affected** - All unimmunized individuals or those with immunizations overdue

   b. **Signs and Symptoms -** Puncture wound, initially muscle stiffness in neck and jaw, progresses to difficulty swallowing and opening mouth, 24 hours after injury all muscles become sensitive to any stimuli, death may result due to respiratory spasm

   c. **Communicable Period** - None

   d. **Seasonal Incidence** - Throughout year

   e. **Transmission** - Inanimate objects, soil, dust, through puncture wounds where spores invade

   f. **Nursing Interventions** - Prevention through updated immunizations; if last immunization was within 5 years, cleanse wound as needed; if last immunization was within 10 years, administer toxoid booster and cleanse wound; if immunization is greater than 10 years old, give toxoid and immunoglobulin and cleanse wound, also monitor for muscle spasms and respiratory status

   g. **Potential Complications** - Pulmonary spasms, laryngospasm, or death

B. Parasitic Infestations

1. **ENTEROBIASIS (PINWORMS)**

   a. **Age Typically Affected** - All ages

   b. **Signs and Symptoms** - Pruritis of anal area, especially at night, may experience anorexia, vulvitis and vaginitis; detected by placing scotch tape over anal opening at night, removing and examining for presence of ova

   c. **Communicable Period** - Anytime child is infected

   d. **Seasonal Incidence** - Throughout year, more common in summer

   e. **Transmission** - Fecal oral route of ova

   f. **Nursing Interventions** - Treat entire family, administer antiparasitic agent as ordered, keep bed linens clean, encourage handwashing

   g. **Potential Complications** - None noted

2. **PEDICULOSIS CAPITIS (HEAD LICE)**

   a. **Age Typically Affected** - Throughout life

   b. **Signs and Symptoms** - Itching of scalp, white balls or salt-like items on hair shaft, especially around nape of neck and behind ears

   c. **Communicable Period** - Anytime eggs present on individual

   d. **Seasonal Incidence** - Throughout year

   e. **Transmission** - Fingernails, shared inanimate objects containing nits such as hairbrushes, combs, hats, bedding, toys

   f. **Nursing Interventions** - Utilize pediculicidal shampoo , such as Kwell, comb out nits, repeat application in 1 week, encourage handwashing, may need to treat entire family, keep linens clean, clean all hair items

   g. **Potential Complications** - Secondary infection due to scratching

3. **SCABIES**

   a. **Age Typically Affected** - All ages

  b. **Signs and Symptoms** - Older children and adolescents: intensely pruritic lesions on anterior axillary lines, inner aspect of upper arm, areolae, penis, wrist, interdigital webs, and ankles; young children: same as older children and adolescents plus palms and soles. Diagnosis based on location of primary lesions, if widespread. If symptoms unclear, lesions are shaved or scraped into a drop of mineral oil and examined microscopically for presence of mites.

  c. **Communicable Period** - Entire time child is infested

  d. **Seasonal Incidence** - Anytime

  e. **Nursing Interventions** - Single application of Lindane lotion from neck down and under fingernails. Infants treated BID with application of 6% sulfur ointment for 3 days. All recently worn clothing and bed linens must be thoroughly laundered and other family members examined and treated as necessary

  f. **Potential Complications** - Infection due to scratching lesions

C. Viral Infections

1. ERYTHEMA INFECTIOSUM (FIFTH'S DISEASE)

  a. **Age Typically Affected** - Children 6 - 10 years

  b. **Signs and Symptoms** - Staged rash: initially begins with mild muscle/joint aches, low-grade fever, sore throat, and headache followed by erythema on face, slapped-cheek appearance (1 - 4 days); progresses to maculopapular rash on all extremities, followed by rash subsiding and becoming lace-like in appearance but reappears with stress, exposure to sunlight, exercise, and temperature changes

  c. **Communicable Period** - Unknown

  d. **Seasonal Incidence** - Most common in winter and spring and occurs in cyclic patterns that peak about every 6 years

  d. **Transmission** - Direct contact by respiratory droplets

  e. **Nursing Interventions** - Supportive of parent and child, infection usually self-limiting

  f. **Potential Complications** - Atypical but may experience arthritic symptoms; children with blood dyscrasias may develop aplastic anemia and should be given immune globulin

2. EXANTHEMA SUBITUM (ROSEOLA)

*Probably viral in origin

  a. **Age Typically Affected** - Children 6 months to 2 years

  b. **Signs and Symptoms** - High fever for 3 - 4 days (103° - 104° F), followed by appearance of macular rash first on trunk then neck, face, and extremities (lasts for 1 - 3 days)

  c. **Communicable Period** - Uncertain

   d. **Seasonal Occurrence** - All year, higher occurrence in spring and fall

   e. **Transmission** - Probably respiratory droplets

   f. **Nursing Interventions** - Assist parents with methods to control fever, discuss seizure precautions and measures, provide parents with information describing this benign infection

   g. **Potential Complications** - Febrile seizures (can be prevented)

4. **MEASLES (RUBEOLA)**

   a. **Age Typically Affected** - Any unimmunized person

   b. **Signs and Symptoms** - Prodromal stage: begins as an upper respiratory infection with fever, malaise, cough, sore throat, Koplik spots, and conjunctivitis. Maculopular rash appears 4 - 5 days after onset of symptoms. Begins on face and spreads to trunk and extremities, rash typically subsides in 3 - 4 days becoming dry and patchy in appearance

   c. **Communicable Period** - 4 days prior to symptoms to 7 days after onset

   d. **Seasonal Occurrence** - Winter and spring

   e. **Transmission** - Respiratory droplets of infected person, or infected inanimate objects contaminated by secretions

   f. **Nursing Interventions** - Treat symptoms as needed, bedrest during initial fever, isolation until noncontagious, fever management, eye care, skin care, maintain hydration, cool humidity for cough

   g. **Potential Complications** - Otitis media, pneumonia, encephalitis, bronchiolitis, myocarditis

5. **MONONUCLEOSIS**

   a. **Age Typically Affected** - Adolescents and young adults

   b. **Signs and Symptoms** - Occur 30 - 50 days following incubation period; headache, anorexia, malaise, extreme fatigue, moderate fever, sore throat, exudate on tonsils, lymphadenopathy, splenomegaly; it is caused by Epstein-Barr virus and has symptoms similar to toxoplasmosis and cytomegalovirus (CMV)

   c. **Communicable Period** - Uncertain

   d. **Seasonal Occurrence** - Throughout year

   e. **Transmission** - Oropharyngeal secretions or intimate contact

   f. **Nursing Interventions** - Comfort measures, bedrest, increase fluids, administer corticosteriods and antibiotics if secondary infections are present

   g. **Potential Complications** - Secondary infections, myocarditis, hemolytic anemia (in severe cases)

6. MUMPS (PAROTITIS)

a. Age Typically Affected - Mainly unimmunized children, all people susceptible

b. Signs and Symptoms - Initially headache, low-grade fever, malaise, anorexia, localized pain around ear and jawline, usually swelling of only one parotid gland, may be quite painful, usually resolves in 3 - 7 days

c. Communicable Period - Uncertain but thought to be before and during swelling phase

d. Seasonal Occurrence - Year-round, more common in winter and spring

e. Transmission - Through saliva of infected person

f. Nursing Interventions - Bedrest, isolation, analgesics, soft diet and increased fluid intake; avoid sour foods

g. Potential Complications - Epidydimo-orchiditis, deafness, encephalitis, myocarditis, hepatitis, neuritis, arthritis, sterility

7. POLIOMYELITIS

a. Age Typically Affected - Any unvaccinated person

b. Signs and Symptoms - May take one of four forms:

- <u>Asymptomatic</u>
- <u>Abortive poliomyelitis</u>: fever, sore throat, headache, abdominal pain, nausea and vomiting
- <u>Nonparalytic poliomyelitis</u>: more severe symptoms as above accompanied by stiffness in back, neck, and legs
- <u>Paralytic poliomyelitis</u>: symptoms as listed in previous forms, progresses to apparent signs of CNS involvement

c. Communicable Period - 3 - 5 days after exposure until 6 - 8 weeks after signs appear

d. Seasonal Incidence - Summer and early fall

e. Transmission - Contact with stool, throat secretions or blood of infected person

f. Nursing Interventions - Treat symptoms as they occur,utilize isolation and enteric precautions, bedrest, PT exercises as indicated, observe paralysis and which systems are affected

g. Potential Complications - Paralysis (temporary or long term), respiratory difficulties

8. RUBELLA (GERMAN MEASLES)

a. Age Typically Affected - Any unimmunized person

b. Signs and Symptoms - May be asymptomatic, low-grade fever, malaise, anorexia, cervical adenopathy, rash appears on face and spreads to trunk and extremities, disappears in same sequence usually within 3 - 4 days

    c. Communicable Period - From 7 days before symptoms to 5 days after rash appears

    d. Transmission - Airborne droplets from respiratory secretions, contaminated articles, feces, urine of infected person

    e. Nursing Interventions - Keep pregnant women in first trimester away from infected child, treat symptoms as needed

    f. Potential Complications - Rare

9. VARICELLA ZOSTER ("CHICKENPOX")

    a. Age Typically Affected - Children 2-8 years of age

    b. Signs and Symptoms - Low-grade fever, rash which progresses from macules, papules, vesicles, and open lesions to scabbing; lesions spread from trunk to extremities and face

    c. Communicable Period - 1 day prior to eruption of lesions until all lesions have scabbed over

    d. Seasonal Incidence - Higher in winter and spring

    e. Transmission - Direct contact with contagious person, respiratory droplets, contaminated inanimate objects

    f. Nursing Interventions - Comfort care to decrease pruritus and secondary infections due to itching; isolate child until scabs have covered all lesions, keep nails short, bathe in baking soda or administer antihistamines and antipruritics to diminish itching sensation

    g. Potential Complications - Scarring, secondary bacterial infections, encephalitis, pneumonia

10

INTEGUMENTARY DISORDERS

I. General Concepts

- The skin functions to regulate heat, provide a means for sensation, protect the body from invading organisms, and prevent desiccation of the underlying structures.

- The skin is composed of the epidermis, dermis, subcutaneous tissues and accessory structures (hair, fingernails, sweat glands, sebaceous glands).

- The skin changes as the infant grows and develops. The epidermis is not adherent to the dermis initially in infancy and this allows for easier blistering. The pH changes from acidic to alkaline with age. Sebaceous glands are active initially at birth then decrease activity until adolescence.

- Skin disorders may be acute or chronic and require treatment to prevent secondary infections.

II. Specific Integumentary Disorder

A. Acquired Disorders

1. ACNE VULGARIS

    a. **Description** - The presence of comedones (blackheads and whiteheads) and pustules that are typically located on the face, chest, and back. It is due to plugging of the sebaceous glands. It is most commonly seen in adolescence as the sebaceous glands become more active.

b. **Signs and Symptoms** - Lesions: blackheads (open comedones), whiteheads (closed comedones), and pustules with inflammation

c. **Diagnostic Procedures** - Diagnosed by characteristic physical findings

d. **Medical Interventions**

  – **Medications** - Application of topical ketolytic (RetinA, Benzoyl peroxide), systemic or topical antibiotic therapy (Tetracycline, Clindamycin), and/or oral retinoids (Accutane)

  – **Treatment** - Focuses on keeping area clean, comedone removal (in some cases), ultraviolet light therapy and estrogen therapy (in some cases)

  – **Surgery** - Unnecessary

e. **Nursing Interventions**

  – **Assessment and Actions**

    • Assess for any areas of inflammation or secondary infection.
    • Discourage vigorous scrubbing or "picking" at the lesions.
    • Assess for signs indicating potential complications.

  – **Teaching**

    • Explain cause and treatment regimen with adolescent and parents.
    • Instruct teen to keep areas clean and to maintain good hygiene in susceptible areas.
    • Instruct teen on avoiding sun exposure after ultraviolet light therapy.
    • Teach parent and teen about medications prescribed (drug, dose, route, and side effects).

  – **Emotional Care**

    • Discuss how teen sees self and promote teens self-esteem.
    • Inform of typical improvement of acne with age.
    • Provide support to family and teen.

f. **Complications** - Scarring, secondary infections

2. ATOPIC DERMATITIS (ECZEMA)

a. **Description** - Superficial dermatitis that occurs in all age groups. It typically begins as pruritic, erythematous, papulovesicular lesions and progresses to crusty, thickened areas. The sites that are frequently affected include cheeks and joints of arms and legs. The etiology is unknown but is thought to be an allergic response. There may be a history of asthma or hayfever in the family.

b. **Signs and Symptoms** - Erythematous, pruritic, papulovesicular lesions followed by scabbing and crust formation in area

c. **Diagnostic Procedures** - Diagnosed by characteristic physical findings

d. **Medical Interventions**

- **Medications** - Administration of antihistamines, antibiotics (systemic), or topical coritcosteroids (Synlar)
- **Treatments** - Focuses on identification of allergen, modification or removal of source of irritation, prevention of secondary infection; application of moist dressings, avoidance of harsh soaps, application of lanolin-based or oil-in-water-based emulsions
- **Surgery** - Unnecessary

e. **Nursing Interventions**

- **Assessment and Actions**
  - Record assessment findings to monitor progress.
  - Assist with determining potential causes and eliminate from environment if possible.
  - Provide method for reducing discomfort.
  - Assess for signs indicating potential complications.
- **Teaching**
  - Explain diagnosis and discuss treatment regimen with family and child.
  - Instruct family on keeping area clean, avoiding hot water to area, taking short baths, applying nonlipid lotions to area, and preventing scratching by using over-the-counter medications, such as diphenhydramine, to diminish pruritus
  - Teach parents about medication prescribed (drug, dose, route, time, and side effects).
- **Emotional Care**
  - Provide support to family and child.

f. **Potential Complications** - Secondary infections, scarring

3. **BURNS**

a. **Description** - Injury to any layer of the skin caused by thermal, chemical or electrical sources.

b. **Signs and Symptoms** - Depend upon severity; superficial-partial thickness burn (first degree: epidermis) exhibits redness and tenderness of area similar to a sunburn; partial thickness burns (second degree: epidermis and dermis with or without appendages affected) exhibit severe pain, area is reddened and may be blistered or dry in appearance; full thickness burns (third degree) are dry, may appear white or leathery and usually lack sensation

c. **Diagnostic Procedures** - Diagnosed by obtaining history of injury and physical findings

d. Medical Interventions

- **Medications** - Application of topical antibiotics and IV antibiotics
- **Treatments** - Treatment depends upon severity, extent and area. Superficial-partial thickness burns are typically treated at home by keeping area cleansed, providing fluids and promoting rest. Partial thickness and full thickness burns are treated by cleaning area several times each day, applying topical antibiotic ointments as ordered, monitoring vital signs, fluid status, urine output, respiratory status, circulation to area; providing pain control, assessing bowel sounds, promoting nutrition, grafting area and providing physical therapy once healed.
- **Surgery** - Escharotomy, skin grafting, or amputation may be necessary

e. Nursing Interventions

- **Assessment and Actions**
  - Obtain vital signs, weight, height and history of injury.
  - Monitor respirations and maintain patent airway especially if injured in closed space or soot present around mouth or nose.
  - Provide method for reducing discomfort.
  - If hospitalization required, monitor: vital signs, airway patency, fluid and electrolyte status, I&O, nutritional intake, circulation to distal area of burn, respiratory status, and bowel sounds; utilize sterile technique for all procedures, document change in wound(s) with each dressing change, position to promote function of injured area (especially joints); place NG tube
  - Administer antibiotics and other medications as ordered.
  - Encourage child to perform own ADLs as able.
  - Facilitate referral (PT, OT, social workers).
  - Assess for signs indicating potential complications.

- **Teaching**
  - Explain injury to parents and child and discuss treatment regimen.
  - If care is to be given at home, teach caregiver how to care for area and about the signs and symptoms which require further medical assistance.
  - If surgery is required, explain procedures to parents and child and plan of care before, during, and after procedure.
  - Ensure proper discharge planning allowing appropriate time for instruction and return demonstration of wound care and physical therapy.
  - Teach parents about medications prescribed (drug, dose, route, time, and side effects).

- **Emotional Care**
  - Encourage parents to be involved with child's care as allowed.
  - Promote growth and development while hospitalized.

- Promote child's self-esteem and discuss change in body and body image.
- Discuss anxiety about treatment and alteration in appearance.
- Provide support to family and child during and after hospitalization.

f. **Potential Complications** - Depend on severity, extent, depth and area of injury but may include infection, contractions, scarring, paralytic ileus, renal failure, shock, acidosis, respiratory failure, loss of limb(s), death

4. CELLULITIS

a. **Description** - An infection of the skin located in the dermis or subcutaneous tissue. It is usually caused by *Staphylococcus aureus*, *Group A beta-hemolytic streptococci*, or *Hemophilus influenza*.

b. **Signs and Symptoms** - Redness, swelling, warmth, induration, and tenderness in area, fever, malaise, lymphangitis; often located in the periorbital area, cheeks, or arms.

c. **Diagnostic Procedures** - Diagnosed by physical findings and history; blood cultures or aspiration may be performed to identify organism; x-ray may be utilized to rule out osteomyelitis.

d. **Medical Interventions**

- **Medications** - Administer organism-specific antibiotic.
- **Treatments** - Apply warm compresses, immobilize area.
- **Surgery** - Unnecessary unless area becomes necrotic

e. **Nursing Interventions**

- **Assessment of Actions**
  - Be alert to signs and symptoms indicating disorder.
  - Monitor and record changes in appearance of skin.
  - If nonresponsive to oral antibiotics, prepare child and family for hospitalization for IV administration.
  - Provide method for reducing discomfort.
  - Assess for signs indicating potential complications.

- **Teaching**
  - Explain diagnosis to parents and child and discuss treatment regimen.
  - Teach parents to keep area immobilized and apply warm soaks to area.
  - Teach parents about medications prescribed (drug, dose, route, time, and side effects).

- **Emotional Care**
  - Provide support to family and child.

f. **Potential Complications** - Systemic infection

5. DIAPER DERMATITIS (DIAPER RASH)

    a. Description - The presence of erythematous lesions and maceration in the diaper area that is due to prolonged contact with urine, feces, or chemical irritants.

    b. Signs and Symptoms - Erythematous lesions which cause discomfort in diaper area

    c. Diagnostic Procedures - Diagnosed by physical findings; rule out fungal and ammoniacal diaper rash which have papules and vesicles

    d. Medical Interventions

       – **Medications** - Apply topical ointments (desitin, A&D, ointments), topical glucocorticoid or if fungal infection is present, application of Nystatin ointment.

       – **Treatments** - Remove irritant, keeping area clean and dry.

       – **Surgery** - Unnecessary

    e. Nursing Interventions

       – **Assessment and Actions**

         • Be alert to signs and symptoms.

         • Provide method for reducing discomfort.

         • Assess for signs indicating potential complications.

       – **Teaching**

         • Explain diagnosis to parents and discuss treatment regimen which includes:

           - Assisting with identifying irritant

           - Discussing importance of keeping area dry and clean

           - Encouraging prompt changing and cleansing of area after each voiding and stool, using mild soap and water

           - Avoiding the use of alcohol-based baby wipes

           - Allowing area to air dry in between changing times

           - Applying ointment to area after cleansed

           - Assessing area with each diaper change for signs of worsening or improvement

           - Discouraging the use of plastic pants

       – **Emotional Care**

         • Provide support to family and reassure infant's irritability will diminish as area heals.

    f. Potential Complications - Discomfort and secondary infections

6. DRUG-INDUCED SKIN REACTION

    a. Description - An allergic reaction to a topical or systemic medication.

    b. Signs and Symptoms - Erythematous and/or urticarial lesions that may be localized or may be widespread depending on route of medication; wheezing; reaction may cause pruritus, fever, and if severe, respiratory distress and anaphylactic shock

   c. **Diagnostic Procedures** - Diagnosed by reviewing history and physical findings

   d. **Medical Interventions**
   - **Medications** - Administer antihistamine and/or corticosteroid; monitor for anaphylactic shock.
   - **Treatments** - Remove or discontinue use of irritant.
   - **Surgery** - Unnecessary

   e. **Nursing Interventions**
   - **Assessment and Actions**
     - Assess child prior to administration of any medication for known allergies and previous response.
     - Observe for signs of reaction and discontinue medication immediately if reaction occurs.
     - Monitor child's vital signs, record reaction symptoms and signs and observe for signs of anaphylactic reaction.
     - Treat pruritus and rash with antihistamines and steroids as ordered.
     - Assess for signs indicating potential complications.
   - **Teaching**
     - Discuss reaction with family and importance of telling future medical teams about reaction.
     - Encourage child to wear a Medic Alert bracelet or tag.
     - Teach parents about reaction, how to prevent and treat.
     - Teach parents about medications prescribed (drug, dose, route, time, and side effects) and when to use.
   - **Emotional Care**
     - Provide support to family and child during treatment regimen.

   f. **Potential Complications** - Anaphylactic reaction

7. **IMPETIGO**

   a. **Description** - A superficial infection of the skin due to invasion by staphylococcal or streptococcal organisms. It typically begins as a scratch that becomes infected. It may be transmitted to others by direct contact with lesion or drainage from lesion. It is usually seen in the infant and toddler age groups and is the most contagious and most common skin infection seen in children.

   b. **Signs and Symptoms** - Begins as erythematous area around dirty scratch; lesion then forms small vesicles that break and release a honey-colored fluid which forms a crust or scab; typically found around mouth, cheeks, face, (especially across the nose) or hands, but may spread over any part of the body

   c. **Diagnostic Procedures** - Diagnosed by characteristic findings and positive culture of vesicular fluid

d. Medical Interventions

- **Medications** - May apply antibacterial ointment, and possibly administer systemic antibiotic therapy (penicillin or dicloxacillin) if
  severe
- **Treatments** - Cleanse area, remove crusts with compresses
  soaked with Burow's solution (astringent solution of aluminum
  acetate)
- **Surgery** - Unnecessary

e. Nursing Interventions

- **Assessment and Actions**
  - Be alert to signs and symptoms.
  - Document appearance, size, and location of lesions.
  - Provide method for reducing discomfort.
  - Assess for signs indicating potential complication.

- **Teaching**
  - Explain diagnosis to parents.
  - Instruct parents on treatment regimen:
    - Cleanse area with Burow's solution as ordered
    - Soak areas that have crusting and scabbing before removal
    - Apply antibacterial ointment as ordered
    - Prevent scratching of area by child
    - If lesions do not improve, discuss need for systemic an-
      tibiotic therapy
    - Emphasize communicability of infection and importance of
      maintaining good hygiene for child and thorough handwash-
      ing for caregiver
    - Teach parents about medications prescribed (drug, dose,
      route, time, and side effects)

- **Emotional Care**
  - Provide support to family and child and reassure that disorder
    can usually be treated at home without complications.

f. Potential Complications - Scarring, acute glomerulonephritis if left
untreated

8. SEBORRHEIC DERMATITIS

a. Description - Erythematous areas of the skin that are due to an excess discharge from the sebaceous glands. It is typically found on the
scalp and eyebrows. It is known as cradle cap in infancy and may also
be present in adolescence.

b. Signs and Symptoms - Patchy lesions on the scalp or eyebrows
which are covered by yellowish, oily scales; area may become
macerated and ooze if left untreated

c. Diagnostic Procedures - Diagnosed by characteristic physical findings

d. Medical Interventions

- **Medications** - Apply mineral oil to infant's scalp, utilize antisebborrheic shampoo, apply topical steroid and/or antibiotics (in some instances).
- **Treatments** - Improve hygiene to area.
- **Surgery** - Not applicable

e. Nursing Interventions

- **Assessment and Actions**
  - Be alert to signs and symptoms indicating disorder.
  - Document appearance, size, and locations of lesions.
  - Determine whether treatment is effective (severe cases may require antiseptic shampoo, topical steroids, and antibiotic therapy).
  - Assess for signs indicating potential complications.

- **Teaching**
  - Discuss treatment regimen with parents and child:
    - Emphasize importance of washing scalp thoroughly with shampoo including the fontanelle in infants (which the parent may be afraid of doing) and rinsing area thoroughly
    - Apply and massage mineral oil on affected area 15 minutes prior to washing infant's scalp to loosen up scales
    - Comb out scales after shampooing

- **Emotional Care**
  - Provide support to parents and child and emphasize that cases are simply treated at home and usually resolve.

f. Potential Complications - Secondary infection to area if left untreated

9. TINEA CAPITIS OR CORPORIS (RINGWORM OF SCALP OR BODY)

a. Description - The presence of a fungal infection on the scalp (tinea capitis) or body (tinea corporis).

b. Signs and Symptoms - Scaly, round or oval erythematous patches on the scalp in areas (capitis) or on the body (corporis); pruritus, and alopecia with broken hair shafts (tinea capitis)

c. Diagnostic Procedures - Diagnosed by utilizing Wood's lamp (sites appear green) and KOH smears (reveals spores)

d. Medical Interventions

- **Medications** - Administer oral griseofulvin, topical antifungals.
- **Treatments** - Frequent shampooing of hair (tinea capitis); keep skin dry and clean (tinea corporis)
- **Surgery** - Unnecessary

e. Nursing Interventions

- **Assessment and Actions**
  - Be alert to signs and symptoms.

- Document appearance, size, and location of lesion.
- Recheck scalp and body after 2 weeks to ensure fungus is gone.
- Assess for signs indicating potential complications.

- **Teaching**
  - Discuss treatment regimen with family and importance of taking/applying medication regularly.
  - Instruct about importance of thorough washing of hair, scalp (tinea capitis) and body every day.
  - Teach parents about medication prescribed (drug, dose, route, time, and side effects).

- **Emotional Care**
  - Discuss alopecia and that hair will grow back in areas once infection treated (tinea capitis).
  - Provide support to family and child.

f. **Potential Complications -** Permanent scarring or baldness if left untreated or treated late (tinea capitis)

11

CENTRAL NERVOUS SYSTEM DISORDERS

I. General Concepts

- The nervous system is comprised of the central nervous system, autonomic nervous system, and peripheral nervous system.

- The nervous system continues to grow and develop after birth and through adolescence.

- The central nervous system (CNS) functions to control and regulate the body. It provides a communication network within the body. It receives information from internal and external stimuli and determines the appropriate response to maintain homeostasis.

II. Specific Central Nervous System Disorders

Congenital Disorders

1. CEREBRAL PALSY

  a. Description - A chronic impairment of motor control and muscle tone resulting from a non-progressive abnormality in the pyramidal motor system. It is often associated with perinatal brain ischemia, prematurity, low birth weight, and birth trauma. There are three major types:
  1) Spastic (comprises majority)
  2) Athetoid
  3) Ataxic

  b. Signs and Symptoms - Depend upon type; general findings include delays and abnormalities in development especially motor control and performance; increased or decreased muscle tone; persistent primitive reflexes; unusual posture; may also exhibit seizure activity, ADD, hyperactivity, mental retardation, and deficits in vision or hearing

  c. Diagnostic Procedures - Usually difficult to diagnose until child is 2-4 months or older when neurological exam reveals abnormalities, including impairment of voluntary muscle movement and posturing

  d. Medical Interventions
  – **Medications** - May administer anticonvulsant and muscle relaxants (diazepam, dantrolene, baclofen) but often benefits do not outweigh side effects
  – **Treatments** - Utilize physical therapy, braces, casts, corrective appliances, glasses, hearing aids
  – **Surgery** - May require surgical correction of spasticity and contractions (including dorsal rhizotomy)

  e. Nursing Interventions
  – **Assessment and Actions**
    • Be alert for signs and symptoms.
    • Monitor child for persistent primitive reflexes; delay in gross motor milestones such as head control, sitting, crawling, feeding difficulties; and failure to develop postural reflexes such as equilibrium.
    • Facilitate referrals to appropriate professional resources (OT, PT) and organizations such as Easter Seals for physical, speech, and occupational therapy, assistance in obtaining special equipment (wheelchairs, car seats).
    • Assess for signs indicating potential complication.
  – **Teaching**
    • Determine parent and child's level of understanding of disorder.

- Teach parent and child about disorder, diagnosis, long-term treatments and implications.
- Assist parent with learning how to care for child and how to enhance growth and development and ADLs.
- Assist parents with determining mode of mobilizing child (wheelchair, braces, walkers), communicating with child, and providing safety for child, including seizure precautions (include provision of safe environment with protection from falls, etc. and may include such interventions as wearing a helmet) and actions to take if seizure occurs.
- Teach parents about medication prescribed (drug, dose, route, time, and side effects).
- Instruct parents on ROM and prevention of skin breakdown.

   – Emotional Care
- Allow for grief response of parents.
   Monitor how family is coping with illness.
- Provide support to family and child.
- Provide support group information to family.

   f. Potential Complications - Delayed growth and development, skin breakdown, contractures, seizures, difficulty with vision, hearing or communicating, may also have various degrees of mental retardation.

2. HYDROCEPHALUS

   a. Description - A problem with over-production, underabsorption or obstruction of flow of CSF in the brain's ventricular circulation. Hydrocephalus may be categorized as communicating or noncommunicating and may be congenital (most common) or acquired.

   b. Signs and Symptoms - Depend upon age; infants: prior to closure of suture lines may exhibit an enlarged head circumference (macrocephaly), bulging fontanels, Macewen's cracked pot sign, setting sun eyes, lethargy, poor feeding, high pitched cry; children may exhibit headaches, vomiting, irritability, seizures, confusion, and a change in level of consciousness, incoordination, papilledema.

   c. Diagnostic Procedures - Diagnosed by physical findings; CT scan reveals enlarged ventricles and site of CSF blockage; x-ray reveals enlarged cranium; MRI may reveal Arnold Chiari malformation (downward displacement of lower brain stem, cerebellum, and fourth ventricle into foramen magnum)

   d. Medical Interventions
   - **Medications** - Administer Isosorbide preoperatively; postoperatively administer acetazolamide, furosemide, antibiotics, anticonvulsant.
   - **Treatments** - Monitor for signs of increased intracranial pressure before and after surgery, ventricular taps in infant (until infant is large enough for shunt placement).

　– **Surgery** - Surgical placement of Ventriculoperitoneal (V-P) or ventricular-atrial (V - A) shunts and removal of obstruction, when possible

e. Nursing Interventions

　– **Assessment and Actions**

　　• Be alert to signs and symptoms that indicate increased intracranial pressure/hydrocephalus.

　　• Monitor infant's head circumference and observe for signs of increasing intracranial pressure (see following section on Increased Intracranial Pressure).

　　• Preoperatively position infant to prevent skin breakdown and support infant's head when turning from side to side.

　　• Postoperatively monitor signs, respiratory and neuro status, maintain adequate hydration and nutrition, assess for signs of IICP and signs of infection, measure I & O carefully.

　　• Assess for signs indicating potential complications.

　– **Teaching**

　　• Explain procedures and treatment regimen to parents and child.

　　• Teach family and child about shunt and how to assess its functioning.

　　• Inform parents and child of signs of shunt malfunction or increased intracranial pressure and when to call physician.

　　• Teach parent to "pump" shunt to assess functioning, if ordered.

　　• Teach child and family that child should be placed on prophylactic antibiotic therapy prior to any dental work or surgical procedure (especially important with V-P shunt).

　– **Emotional Care**

　　• Promote growth and development.

　　• Provide support to family and child.

　　• Provide support group information to family.

f. Potential Complications - Infection, obstruction or malfunction of shunt, subdural hematoma, infection or perforation of abdominal contents after placement. Death will occur if IICP is not detected or left untreated.

3. NEURAL TUBE DEFECT

a. Description - The failure of the neural plate to close posteriorly in the midline. The most frequently seen defect is a myelomeningocele, a congenital defect where the spinal cord contents protrude through the spinal column in an enclosed sac-like structure. There are three major types: anencephaly (little or absent brain tissue; incompatible with life), encephalocele (midline defect in skull containing protruding cranial contents), myelodysplasia or spina bifida (malformation of vertebral column, meninges, and spinal cord).

b. **Signs and Symptoms** - Visual observation of defect; may have associated neurological defects such as loss of bladder and bowel control, and paraplegia. A less severe form of spina bifida (spina bifida occult) appears as a dimple on the lower sacral area but on further investigation it is noncystic and does not contain contents of the spinal cord.

c. **Diagnostic Procedures** - Diagnosed by physical findings, neurological exam determines level of defect; x-ray, MRI, CT scan, and ultrasound reveal spinal cord involvement and associated abnormalities such as hydrocephalus

d. **Medical Interventions**

   – **Medications** - Administer antibiotics (pre- and postoperatively), oxybutynin chloride (Ditropan), propantheline, stool softeners, laxatives, anticonvulsant, antispasmodics (for hypertonic bladder), choleric agents (for hypotonic bladder).

   – **Treatments** - Utilize correct positioning, maintain bowel and bladder care.

   – **Surgery** - Surgical closure of defect is performed shortly after birth; continent ileal reservoir or urinary diversion may be necessary.

e. **Nursing Interventions**

   – **Assessment and Actions**

     • Assess newborn thoroughly for sign of defect.

     • Protect sac covering preoperatively, keep sac moist with sterile gauze, place infant in heated environment, position infant in prone or side-lying position, avoid diapering; post operatively: assess vital signs, hydration, level of comfort, nutrition, and place in prone- or side-lying position, also monitor for increased intracranial pressure, signs of infection, place "donut" under head if V-P shunt placed to decrease pressure on shunt reservoir.

     • Assess for signs indicating potential complications (infection, IICP, seizures).

   – **Teaching**

     • Explain diagnosis to family and treatment regimen.

     • Provide information regarding ROM exercises, positioning, mobilization devices, bladder and bowel elimination, and skin care.

     • Assist family with planning care for child once discharged.

   – **Emotional Care**

     • Promote child's growth and development.

     • Provide support to family and child.

     • Provide support group information to family.

    f. Potential Complications - Disorder may also be accompanied by hydrocephalus, genitourinary disorders, paralysis; decubitus ulcers, dislocation of hips, delay in development, stress in family, bladder infections, meningitis, injury and infection of lower extremities

Acquired Disorders

1. BACTERIAL MENINGITIS

    a. Description - An infection and inflammation of the meninges (coverings) of the brain usually due to *Hemophilus influenza* (type B), *Streptococcus pneumonia* or *Neisseria meningitidis*. Neonatal meningitis is most often caused by *E. coli.* It may result from otitis media or sinusitis. It can be fatal.

    b. Signs and Symptoms - Depends upon organism, severity, and age of child; infants have vague and various signs and symptoms: headache, irritability, fever, seizure, drowsiness, poor feeding, vomiting, stiff neck, positive Kernig and Brudzinski signs, petechiae

    c. Diagnostic Procedures - Diagnosed by positive lumbar puncture (LP), positive blood culture, elevated spinal fluid pressure and elevated WBC. If IICP suspected, CT scan may be ordered. If IICP confirmed, LP not performed to diminish risk of cranial herniation from sudden decrease in ICP.

    d. Medical Interventions

        – **Medications** - Administer antibiotic therapy appropriate for organism, anticonvulsant, antipyretics, electrolyte replacement.

        – **Treatments** - Monitor and relieve increased intracranial pressure and cerebral edema, monitor hydration and electrolyte status, and replace as necessary.

        – **Surgery** - Unnecessary

    e. Nursing Interventions

        – **Assessment and Action**

            • Maintain (Hib) immunizations up-to-date to prevent contraction of *H. influenzae.*

            • Be alert for signs indicating disorder.

            • Maintain medication therapy, hydration.

            • Monitor neurological and respiratory status and provide quiet environment.

            • Maintain respiratory body fluid isolation status.

            • Provide method for reducing discomfort.

            • Assess for signs indicating potential complications.

            • Provide relief from fever with medications, tepid baths, cooling blanket.

        – **Teaching**

            • Explain procedures and treatment to family.

- Teach family importance of isolation and seizure control.
- Teach family about medications prescribed (drug, dose, route, time, and side effects).
  - **Emotional Care**
    - Provide support to family and child.
    - Provide support group information.
- **f. Potential Complication** - If treated promptly, uncommon; may experience disseminated intravascular coagulation (DIC) syndrome of inappropriate antidiuretic hormone secretion (SIADH), hydrocephalus, peripheral circulatory collapse, permanent neurological impairment, death

2. ENCEPHALITIS

- **a. Description** - An inflammation or infection of the brain resulting in swelling, cellular damage and temporary or permanent neurological dysfunction. It is most commonly caused by viral agents but may be bacterial or fungal in origin or result from toxins such as arsenic or lead.
- **b. Signs and Symptoms** - Headache, lethargy, drowsiness, disturbance in speech, language, motor skills; seizures, change in level of consciousness, malaise, fever, dizziness, stiffness of neck, nausea, vomiting. Onset may be gradual or rapid depending on cause.
- **c. Diagnostic Procedures** - Diagnosed by physical findings, positive culture from lumbar puncture and Gram stain
- **d. Medical Intervention**
  - **Medications** - Administer antibiotics according to causative agent, steroids, osmotic diuretics, electrolyte replacement, anticonvulsant, antidotes to identified toxins
  - **Treatment** - Supportive care and monitoring for complications
  - **Surgery** - Unnecessary
- **e. Nursing Interventions**
  - **Assessment and Actions**
    - Monitor neuro status, vital signs, and provide comfort measures (dim lights, limit noise).
    - Facilitate appropriate referrals as necessary (speech therapy, OT, PT).
    - Assess for signs indicating potential complications (seizures, permanent neuro impairment, death).
  - **Teaching**
    - Assess parents' level of understanding.
    - Discuss with parents and child procedures and treatment regimen allowing for questions.
    - Prepare parents and child for home care.

- Teach parents about medication prescribed (drug, dose, route, time, and side effects).
  - **Emotional Care**
    - Encourage parents to visit child or remain with child while hospitalized.
    - Discuss the impact the neurological deficits, if present, have on parent and child.
    - Provide support to parents and child.
    - Provide support group information to family.
  f. **Potential Complications** - Residual neurological deficits, delay in meeting developmental tasks, death

3. REYE'S SYNDROME

  a. **Description** - A toxic invasion of the brain accompanied by severe cerebral edema, liver enlargement and fatty infiltration. It most commonly follows a viral infection and has been associated with the ingestion of aspirin. It most commonly occurs in males and has a high morality rate.

  b. **Signs and Symptoms** - Initially has signs similar to common cold; then child appears to be well, followed by vomiting, hyperpnea, irregular respirations, dilated sluggish pupil reaction, and nervous system dysfunctions, neurological signs continue to progress from disorientation to various stages of coma; liver dysfunction and unresponsiveness follow

  c. **Diagnostic Procedures** - Diagnosed by history of prodromal respiratory infection, influenza A or B, or chicken pox; presence of elevated AST (formerly SGOT) and ALT (formerly SGPT), LDH, bilirubin, and PTT; decreased serum glucose in children less than 5 years and hyperglycemia and pancreatitis in older children; abnormalities in EEG, increased serum ammonia

  d. **Medical Interventions**
    - **Medications** - Administer mannitol, insulin, vitamin K for clotting disturbances, anticonvulsant, and possibly barbiturates.
    - **Treatments** - Treatment depends upon stage of illness but includes:
      Stage 1 - Maintain serum glucose level and reduce cerebral edema via IV fluids.
      Stages 2 - 5 - Reduce ICP, mannitol administration, tracheal intubation to control blood pH.
    - **Surgery** - Unnecessary

  e. **Nursing Interventions**
    - **Assessment and Action**
      - Be alert to signs and symptoms.
      - Monitor vital signs, ICP, cerebral edema, fluid status.

- Assess for signs indicating potential complications.
  - **Teaching**
    - Provide information on prevention of disorder including discouraging parents from utilizing aspirin during a child's illness.
    - Discuss with parents diagnosis, treatments, and allow parents to ask questions.
  - **Emotional Care**
    - Provide support to family and child.
    - Provide support group information to family.
  - **f. Potential Complications** - Neurological deficits, aspiration pneumonitis, respiratory failure, death

4. SEIZURE DISORDERS

- **a. Description** - Seizures are transient alterations in brain functioning resulting from overproduction of disorganized electrical charges and are manifested as alterations in level of consciousness or motor, sensory or autonomic functioning. They may be due to either congenital or acquired defects. They are categorized according to the cause and location of the neuronal discharge. Most seizures are idiopathic in nature.

- **b. Signs and Symptoms** - Depend upon site of abnormal neurological discharge
  - **Categories Include:**
    - **Partial seizures** - One hemisphere of the brain is usually affected
      - Complex partial seizures: Psychomotor seizures in which motor movement occurs without child's awareness (smacking, speaking, repetitive movement), child is amnesic of events, usually preceded by odor, taste, or sensation ("aura") and followed by sleep episode and postictal symptoms
      - Simple partial seizures: Involuntary autonomic, sensory or motor function with child usually remaining conscious
    - **Generalized seizures** - Both hemispheres of the brain are affected
      - Absence seizures - Traditionally known as petit mal seizures; lapse in consciousness without associated movement; often seizure is unnoticed, may be mistaken for daydreaming
      - Atonic and akinetic seizures - Inability to maintain posture and inability to move; sudden uncontrollable drop attacks with brief loss of consciousness
      - Infantile spasms - Assumes flexed neck, drawn up legs and extended arms posture without loss of consciousness; often followed by crying or cooing (3 - 12 months

typical age); disappears with age and often replaced by other type of seizure; associate with brain abnormality

· Myoclonic seizures - Muscle contraction followed by relaxation (single muscle group); child remains conscious

· Tonic clonic seizures - Traditionally known as grand mal seizures; contraction of muscles followed by jerking movement and relaxation: often exhibits cyanosis during contraction phase, bowel and bladder incontinence; child is unconscious during seizure

- **Other**

  · Febrile seizure - Tonic clonic seizure due to extreme rise (usually >102°F or 39°C) in temperature, usually occurs only once during febrile episode, if fever brought under control it usually is without lasting effects

  · Status epilepticus - Repetitive tonic clonic seizure without regaining consciousness between episodes; Emergency - respiratory failure and death can ensue

c. **Diagnostic Procedures** - Diagnosed by identifying cause and may include: CBC, lumbar puncture, X-ray, CT scan; screening for TORCH (T-Toxoplasmosis, O-Other [such as hepatitis], R-Rubella, C-Cytomegalovirus, H-Herpes simplex); video monitored EEG to identify behavior associated with seizure, brain mapping

d. **Medical Interventions**
   - **Medications** - Administer anticonvulsant.
   - **Treatments** - Treatment depends upon cause and type of seizure but requires anticonvulsant therapy and providing safety for child.
   - **Surgery** - Surgical interventions may be necessary to diminish or eliminate the uncontrolled neuronal firing.

e. **Nursing Interventions**
   - **Assessment and Actions**
     · Obtain detailed and thorough history.
     · Be alert to signs and symptoms that indicate seizure disorder.
     · Assess seizure and monitor if certain events precede or follow.
     · Document seizures (onset, duration, pattern of movements, recovery).
     · Maintain safe environment and utilize precautions.
     · Assess vital signs and neurological status of child.
     · Record serum level of anticonvulsant and monitor for side effects of medication.
     · Assess for signs indicating potential complications.
   - **Teaching**
     · Teach parents and child about disorder, its cause and about treatment regimen; allow questions and explain on a level that a child can understand.

- Inform parents about importance of seizure precautions and how to assist child during seizures (assist to floor, do not restrain, monitor breathing, do not force something into mouth, protect from injury, remove tight clothing, comfort child afterwards).
- Teach parents about medication prescribed (drug, dose, route, time, and side effects).
- Teach necessity of returning for follow-up visits/care and for drug level testing.
- Stress importance of good dental hygiene if taking phenytoin.
  - **Emotional Care**
    - Determine parent's and child's level of coping with disorder.
    - Assess anxiety level of parents and child.
    - Promote growth and development and enhance child's self esteem.
    - Provide support to family and child.
    - Provide support group information to family.
  f. **Potential Complications** - Injury during seizures; numerous side effects from medications (behavior changes, bleeding problems, liver and kidney changes); possible drug toxicity; death (if respiratory failure occurs)

Sensory Disorders

1. AUDITORY DISTURBANCES

a. **Description** - The temporary or permanent loss of conductive, central auditory, sensorineural, or mixed sensorineural hearing. Hearing deficits are one of most common disabilities in childhood and range from slight to extreme hearing loss.

b. **Signs and Symptoms** - Vary; may find a diminished startle reflex and low score for response to human voice on Brazelton Neonatal Assessment in neonates; difficulty in learning, speech delay or delay in response to voice; increased visual attention, diminished response to verbal directions; behavior problems or withdrawn behavior.

c. **Diagnostic Procedures** - Audiometry reveals diminished or absent hearing, tympanometry reveals decreased movement, brainstem auditory evoked potentials show decreased brain potential. Rinne and Weber tests are negative.

d. **Medical Interventions**
  - **Medications** - Administer antibiotics if infection is present.
  - **Treatments** - Treatment depends on cause and severity of loss, but ranges from hearing aids to surgical implants or corrections.
  - **Surgery** - May require surgical implant or tube placement.

  e. **Nursing Interventions**
    – **Assessment and Actions**
      • Be alert for signs and symptoms that indicate a hearing loss.
      • Prevent by keeping child's immunizations current, monitoring or reducing loud noises in the environment, appropriately treating otitis media.
      • Notify school nurse/teachers, other parents, and friends of deficit and how to communicate.
      • Facilitate referral (speech therapy, audiology).
      • Assess for signs indicating potential complications.
    – **Teaching**
      • Explain to parent and child significance and duration of loss.
      • Provide information on diagnosis, treatment and methods of coping with deficit: use of hearing aid, sign language, lip reading, speech therapy, ways to enhance child's growth and development.
    – **Emotional Care**
      • Promote growth and development and socialization.
      • Provide support to family and child.
      • Provide support group information to family.
  f. **Potential Complications** - Potential for delay in development and socialization

2. **VISUAL DISTURBANCES**
  a. **Description** - Any alteration in vision. It may be due to a variety of factors and may be congenital (cataracts, glaucoma), or acquired. The disturbance may be categorized as an acute or chronic disorder. It may range from slight impairment to complete impairment.

  b. **Signs and Symptoms** - Depend on type and severity; may have poor motor control of eyes (strabismus), diminished vision in one eye (amblyopia), visual opaqueness in lens (cataract), increased intraocular pressure (glaucoma), visible wound or abnormality of eye (trauma or malformation), inability to make eye contact or follow objects, may not reach for items, may bump into things, or complain of inability to see, may show a delay in fine and gross motor skills as development continues, may exhibit poor school work, frequently rub eyes or squint, exhibit poor peripheral vision

  c. **Diagnostic Procedures** - Diagnosed by finding abnormalities in the following tests: Neonatal Brazelton Assessment Scoring, visual assessment with and without ophthalmoscope, funduscopic examination, vision screening (Snellen chart)

  d. **Medical Interventions**
    – **Medications** - May require miotic therapy, anticholinesterase, or antibiotics (if infection present)

- **Treatments** - Depend on cause and severity of visual disturbance; may require correction with lenses or patching of eye
- **Surgery** - Corrective surgery may be necessary for persistent strabismus, cataracts, glaucoma, or foreign body removal

e. **Nursing Interventions**
- **Assessment and Actions**
  - Screen children at early age and detect abnormalities.
  - Monitor child's ability to perform ADLs.
  - Provide safe environment if hospitalized.
  - Familiarize child with environment.
  - Introduce self and speak to child when entering or exiting room.
  - Assess for signs indicating potential complications.
- **Teaching**
  - Provide anticipatory guidance by making parent and child aware of safety needs of eyes.
  - Explain findings of eye exam to parent and child.
  - Provide education for parents according to necessary treatment: necessity of glasses or lenses and proper care, instillation of eye drops (drug, dose, times, and side effects), care of prosthesis.
  - Prepare child and family for surgical correction as appropriate and what to expect before, during and after surgery.
  - Teach parents how to interact with child if impairment is severe and permanent (familiarize child with environment and don't change it suddenly, promote bonding, enhance development, encourage independence, provide safety for child, assist with schooling and inform teachers of child's special needs).
- **Emotional Care**
  - Discuss impact diagnosis has on child and family.
  - Promote growth, development and socialization.
  - Provide support to family and child.
  - Provide support group information to family.

f. **Potential Complications** - Delay in growth and development, postoperative infection, injury due to visual deficit

Disorders Arising from Trauma

1. COMA

a. **Description** - A temporary or permanent alteration in alertness or consciousness in which the child is not aroused with even strong stimulus. It may include: unresponsiveness to specific stimuli, absence of reflexes, lack of spontaneous breathing, and flat EEG. It may be the result of a variety of cerebral insults and may be categorized from light coma to brain death.

b. **Signs and Symptoms** - Altered or abnormal neurological scoring in relation to eye opening, motor and verbal response using a pediatric coma scale or Glasgow Coma scale

c. **Diagnostic Procedures** - Diagnosed by physical findings; diagnosis procedures utilized depend on causative factor but may include culture and sensitivity to rule out organisms; evaluation of blood oxygen levels to rule out hypoxia; lumbar puncture to rule out organisms and cancerous diagnosis, EEG to determine brain activity; and CT scan to determine if mass is present; urinalysis to determine if toxin present

d. **Medical Interventions**
   - **Medications** - Medications given according to causative factor or to treat possible complications and may include corticosteroids, barbiturates, diuretics
   - **Treatments** - Maintain vital functions, monitor ICP and neurological status, monitor for and treat complications.
   - **Surgery** - May be necessary if due to pressure or mass in brain

e. **Nursing Interventions**
   - **Assessment and Actions**
     - Assess child's neurological status as ordered noting changes.
     - Monitor vital signs, respiratory status, hydration, nutrition, bowel and bladder functioning, and skin temperature and intactness.
     - Document neuro status as ordered.
     - Assess for signs indicating potential complications.
     - If appropriate discuss brain death and potential organ donation.
   - **Teaching**
     - Discuss diagnosis and treatment regimen with parents, allowing for questions.
     - Provide information regarding safety of child to prevent head injuries, near drownings, or other trauma that may lead to neurological insults leading to comatose state.
     - Teach parents how to care for child (feeding, bathing, exercising, turning).
   - **Emotional Care**
     - Speak to child during procedures.
     - Provide support to parents and assess coping level.
     - Provide support group information to parents.

f. **Potential Complications** - Skin breakdown, contractures (if longterm) respiratory or bladder infections, residual neurological damage, and death

2. HEAD INJURY

a. Description - An open or closed injury to the cranium and its contents resulting from mechanical force. The term head injury includes concussions, contusions, skull fractures, vascular injuries, and cerebral edema. The prognosis depends on the extent of the injury.

b. Signs and Symptoms - Depend on severity but include: headache, loss of consciousness, bradycardia, hypotension, CSF leakage from an orifice, vomiting, irritability, increased intracranial pressure, seizures

c. Diagnostic Procedures - Diagnosed by physical findings; diagnostic tests utilized depend on history of injury but may include the following: skull X-ray may show damage, EEG may exhibit alteration, CT scan may show bleeding, cerebral angiography reveals hemorrhaging

d. Medical Interventions

  – **Medications** - Administer antibiotics if open injury present; may require osmotic diuretics if cerebral swelling present; may administer anticonvulsants.

  – **Treatments** - Depend on severity of injury but may include home observation, monitoring airway, treating for shock, aspiration of fluid, monitoring of vital signs and ICP.

  – **Surgery** - Surgical intervention may be necessary if hemorrhaging is present or cranium is fractured or crushed

e. Nursing Interventions

  – **Assessment and Actions**

  • Always assume child has cervical and spinal injuries until ruled out.

  • Be alert to signs and symptoms that may indicate injury.

  • Maintain airway and stabilize head and neck.

  • Obtain a careful history if head injury suspected.

  • Assess vital signs and level of consciousness frequently.

  • Be alert for signs of contrecoup injuries (signs of internal injury on the side opposite the direct injury to the head).

  • If hospitalization is required, monitor vital signs, neuro status, including reflexes and level of consciousness, maintain bedrest, keep environment quiet, assess for any drainage from ears or nose, periorbital ecchymosis (raccoon eyes), postauricular ecchymosis (Battle sign), observe for signs of increased intracranial pressure, assess for other injuries, provide only clear liquids until stable and alert.

  • Assess for signs of child maltreatment syndrome (CMS).

  • Assess for signs indicating potential complications.

- **Teaching**
  - Provide anticipatory guidance to parents by informing them of the higher risk of head injuries in children and suggest ways to diminish injury.
  - Discuss with parents diagnoses and treatment regimen, if home care needed, teach parents to observe for abnormal signs and symptoms (change in level of consciousness and/or in pupils, presence of double vision, change in coordination) and when to contact the physician.
- **Emotional Care**
  - Provide support to family and child.
  - Provide support group information to family.

f. **Potential Complications** - Infection, neurological deficits, coma, death

3. INCREASED INTRACRANIAL PRESSURE

a. **Description** - An increase in the normal pressure of the CSF. It may be caused by excess production of CSF, obstruction of flow of CSF, or increased size of brain mass, (due to swelling, injury, infection or tumors).

b. **Signs and Symptoms** - Depend upon age; infants (before suture lines close) enlarged head circumference, bulging fontanels, setting sun eyes, high-pitched cry, poor feeding; children: headache, vomiting, irritability, change in level of consciousness, drowsiness, poor attention span; as pressure increases signs may include: change in vital signs, loss of consciousness, change in pupils, altered or clumsy movements; change in posturing (decerebrate or decorticate posture), seizures, respiratory arrest.

c. **Diagnostic Procedures** - Diagnosed by physical findings, CSF reveals increased pressure, CT scan and MRI reveal mass or blockage, EEG may reveal decreased activity

d. **Medical Interventions**
   - **Medications** - Administer osmotic diuretics (Mannitol), restrict fluids, and administer steroids, barbiturates, antacids, barbiturates, cimetidime or ranitidime, antacids, antipyretics.
   - **Treatments** - Monitor vital signs, respiratory and neurological status, IICP monitoring by subarachnoid bolt, hyperventilation (to decrease $PaCO_2$ and increase PaO_2 thereby decreasing cerebral edema).
   - **Surgery** - Surgical correction by removal of mass, stopping hemorrhaging, or opening passageway for flow of CSF production, V-P or V-A shunt placement, extraventricular drain (EVD) placement

   e. **Nursing Interventions**
      - **Assessment and Actions**
         • Be alert to signs of IICP.
         • Monitor IICP, VS, respiratory functioning, neuro status (including subtle changes in level of consciousness, personality, and motor function); elevate head of bed 30-45 degrees and keep head in neutral alignment, avoid flexion of neck; keep environment quiet.
         • Monitor fluid status and nutrition.
         • Administer medications as ordered.
         • Assess for signs indicating potential complications.
      - **Teaching**
         • Explain to family diagnosis and treatment regimen.
         • Teach parents about medication prescribed (drug, dose, route, time and side effects).
      - **Emotional Care**
         • Provide support to family and child.
         • Provide support group information to family.
   f. **Potential Complications** - Infection, neurological deficits, respiratory failure, death

Other

1. **ATTENTION DEFICIT HYPERACTIVITY DISORDER (ADHD)**

   a. **Description** - The inability to control attention span, impulses, and activity level that is appropriate for age. It is a type of learning disability of unknown etiology. It is more commonly seen in males. It appears to be a genetic component, as well as, associated with maternal alcohol abuse and metabolic and/or infectious diseases during childhood.

   b. **Signs and Symptoms** - Depends on severity but may include inability to maintain attention level, exhibition of hyperactivity, inability to delay impulses, easily frustrated, inability to complete a task; symptoms usually present before 7 years of age and have lasted at least 6 months

   c. **Diagnostic Procedures** - Diagnosed by reviewing history and descriptive report by parents and teachers, utilizing psychological screening, EEG may reveal abnormal findings, CT scan may show mild cerebral atrophy

   d. **Medical Interventions**
      - **Medications** - Administer methylphenidate, dextroamphetamine, or pemoline (Ritalin, Dexedrine or Silar).
      - **Treatment** - May require psychotherapy or behavior modification.
      - **Surgery** - Unnecessary

e. Nursing Interventions

– Assessment and Actions

- Be alert to signs and symptoms of ADHD.
- Network with school nurse and teachers.
- Monitor factors causing exacerbations (foods, environment, time of day).
- Facilitate appropriate referral (behavior therapist).
- Assess for signs indicating potential complications.

– Teaching

- Explain disorder and treatment regimen to parents and child.
- Discuss medication therapy and potential side effects.
- Assist parent with behavior therapy and reducing environmental stimulation.

– Emotional Care

- Discuss impact disorder has on child and family.
- Promote growth and development, as well as, healthy social interaction.
- Provide support to family and child.
- Provide support group information to family.

f. Potential Complications - Medication side effects may produce growth retardation or delay in developmental level; developmental delay may be prevented by decreasing the dose of the medication or stopping the medication periodically.

12

ONCOLOGY DISORDERS

I. General Concepts

- Cancer is defined as the occurrence and overproduction of abnormal cells.

- Cancer may develop in any tissue.

- The cause of cancer is unknown but may be related to genetics, the environment, and nutritional intake.

- Cancer is categorized according to its level of development and sites where metastasis has occurred.

- Cardinal signs and symptoms of most cancers include: pain, anorexia, weight loss, change in behavior, frequent infection, bleeding episodes, fever, and open sore(s) that will not heal.

- Cancer is considered to be cured if the tumor does not occur within 5 years of completing treatment.

II. Specific Treatments

* Regimens for malignant tumors typically follow specific protocols for the particular cancerous cells but may include the following:

Bone Marrow Transplants

The placement of healthy bone marrow into a diseased area. It may be retrieved from an allogenic (related or unrelated donor), autologous (donor and recipient are the same), or a syngeneic donor (donor and recipient are identical twins). It requires long-term hospitalization, immunosuppression prior to and after transplantation and isolation. Complications include infection and graft vs. host disease (GVHD).

Chemotherapy

The administration of antineoplastic agents*. It may be used as the only treatment or may be combined with other therapies. The placement of a long-term catheter for drug administration is required (Port or Broviac). Chemotherapy is classified according to the action of the drug and may include the use of the following categories:

1. **Alkylating Agents**: Chlorambucil, Cyclophosphamide, Mechlorethamine
2. **Antibiotics:** Actinomycin -D, Bleomycin, Daunorubicin, and Doxorubicin
3. **Antimetabolites:** 5-Azacytidine, Cytosine arabinoside, Mercaptopurine, Methotrexate, and 6-Thioguanine
4. **Enzymes:** L-asparaginases
5. **Hormones:** Corticosteroids
6. **Plant Alkaloids**: Vincristine and Vinblastine
7. **Others**: Cisplatin, Dacarbazine, Hydroxyurea, and Procarbazine

* Each agent has specific side effects. The most commonly seen reactions include nausea, vomiting, anorexia, alopecia, stomatitis, diarrhea, abdominal pain, dermatitis, weight loss. Extremely high doses may affect the heart and nervous system.

Immunotherapy

The stimulation of the body's immune response through administration of medications or immunoglobulins

Palliative Therapy

Treatments which provide comfort and relieve pain or pressure. These treatments are not intended to cure. It includes the reduction of side effects of medication or treatments, the surgical removal of the tumor to decrease discomfort, and the administration of analgesics or narcotics.

Radiotherapy

The administration of ionizing radiation to the diseased area. The side effects depend upon the location that is being treated but include nausea, vomiting, diarrhea, GI ulceration, alopecia, dermatitis, cystitis, and anemia.

Surgical Removal

The excision of all or part of the diseased area. It may be a curative or palliative procedure or assist in slowing the growth process of the tumor.

III. General Nursing Interventions

Assessment and Actions

1. Be alert to signs and symptoms of cancer.
2. Diminish potential for infection by maintaining isolation.
3. Monitor vital signs and I&O during drug administration.
4. Assess infusion site carefully for signs of extravasation and stop infusion and notify MD immediately if infiltration occurs.
5. Promote nutrition by offering foods requested, offering small meals and mild-flavored food, avoid offering favorite foods during periods of nausea, providing mouth care, decreasing offensive odors in room or environment,administering antiemetics before meals may also help, applying anesthetics to ulcers in mouth and monitoring weight daily.
6. Encourage activity as tolerated, including rest periods each day.
7. Provide therapy for potential neuropathies as they occur: foot drop, jaw pain, difficulty walking.
8. Provide for comfort by repositioning, using gentle massage, warmth, cold application, analgesic administration
9. Assess for signs indicating potential complications (specific to medications or location of tumor).

Teaching

1. Prepare child and family for diagnostic procedures by explaining type of procedure and preparations that are necessary before and after procedure.
2. Explain diagnosis and discuss treatment regimen.
3. Assess family and child's level of understanding.
4. Instruct family and child on methods for reducing discomfort.

5. Instruct family and child on importance of preventing exposure of child to infection.

6. Teach family and child how to select foods which will increase protein in take and to avoid foods which may cause nausea.

7. Prepare child and family for procedures and treatments by providing appropriate information on what to expect before, during, and after each necessary activity (bone marrow aspiration, lumbar puncture, medication administration, port or catheter placement).

8. Teach parents and child about medication prescribed (drug, dose, route, and side effects).

9. Discuss long-term care needs as appropriate.

10. Prepare parents and child for discharge.

11. Teach parents and child to prevent contact with others who are sick while immunocompromised.

Emotional Care

1. Promote child's growth and development while being treated by enhancing independence with activities appropriate for age.

2. Provide family with an environment which allows questions and concerns to be considered and answered.

3. Discuss with child and family how disease is impacting lifestyle.

4. Discuss with child how he is adapting to change in body image.

5. Assist child with adapting to loss of body part or change in body appearance.

6. Provide honest information, do not give false reassurance.

7. Be prepared to discuss death with parent or child and listen to concerns or beliefs.

8. Provide emotional support to family and child.

9. Provide support group information to family and child.

10. Allow for grieving and anger, assure child and family that this is part of the grieving process.

IV. Specific Oncology Disorders

1. BRAIN TUMORS

   a. **Description** - Abnormal tissue growth within the cranium. It may be infratentorial or supratentorial in location. It is categorized according to the tissue that is affected. The most common brain tumors in the pediatric population are gliomas. The survival rate for brain tumors ranges from 20% to 77% depending upon the location and response of the tumor to treatment.

   b. **Signs and Symptoms** - Depend on upon age of child, anatomical location and size of tumor; child may not exhibit signs until late in disease process if suture lines of skull are not closed; findings include headache and vomiting especially after arising in the morning, dizziness, irritability, drowsiness, change in motor control, weakness, failure to thrive, change in level of consciousness or behavior, altered vision, change in vital signs, seizures, nuchal rigidity

c. **Diagnostic Procedures** - Diagnosed by reviewing history and abnormal physical findings especially in neurological status; CT scan allows for visualization of mass, angiography shows vascular supply to tumor, MRI reveals location and size of mass, intracranial biopsy determines whether mass is benign or malignant

d. **Medical Interventions**
   – **Medications** - Administer chemotherapy according to specific protocol.
   – **Treatments** - Administer radiation therapy.
   – **Surgery** - Surgical excision of tumor if possible.

e. **Nursing Interventions** - (See previous list of General Nursing Interventions)
   – **Assessment and Actions**
     • Preoperatively monitor child's vital signs and neuro status.
     • Postoperatively monitor vital signs, fluid status, neuro status; position patient with head in midline and elevate head of bed as ordered; keep environment as quiet as possible; provide method for reducing discomfort.
   – **Teaching**
     • Prepare child and family for treatment regimen by describing what to expect before, during, and after surgical procedure.
     • Explain side effects of chemotherapy and radiation therapy and how to reduce side effects.
     • Discuss long-term therapy that is necessary after discharge.
   – **Emotional Care**
     • Do not provide false hope but be honest with family and child.
     • Encourage family to continue routine life at home as much as possible.
     • Provide suggestions for alternatives for covering head after surgery to promote child's body image.

f. **Potential Complications** - Neurological impairment (paralysis, visual or auditory impairment, coma, seizures - depends on area of brain affected or removed), infection, delays in growth and development, and death

2. EWING'S SARCOMA

a. **Description** - A tumor of the bone marrow. It usually affects the long bones and bones of the trunk. It is a highly malignant tumor.

b. **Signs and Symptoms** - Bone pain and discomfort, swelling in affected area

c. Diagnostic Procedures - Diagnosed by physical findings, bone marrow aspiration reveals abnormal cells, x-ray reveals bone destruction, and surgical biopsy confirms diagnosis and whether tumor is benign or malignant

d. Medical Interventions

- **Medications** - Administer chemotherapy according to specific protocol.
- **Treatment** - Administer radiation therapy to area.
- **Surgery** - Surgical excision of affected area or possibly amputation

e. Nursing Interventions - (See previous list of General Nursing Interventions)

- **Assessment and Actions**
  - Preoperatively monitor vital signs and provide methods for reducing discomfort.
  - Postoperatively monitor vital signs, site for hemorrhaging, elevate amputation above level of the heart, monitor I&O, and provide method for reducing pain (administer analgesics antienflammatous, narcotics as ordered).
  - Assist with returning child to ambulatory status as soon as possible.
- **Teaching**
  - Explain effects of treatment and ways to relieve discomfort.
  - Explain that use of extremity need not be limited.
  - Prepare family and child for long-term treatment regimen.
  - If surgical resection or amputation is necessary, explain treatment, allow for questions and concerns to be addressed.
  - Teach crutch-walking and placement and use of prosthesis as necessary.
- **Emotional Care**
  - Promote return to normal lifestyle as soon as possible.
  - Support family and child during time of grieving.
  - Discuss with child the impact disorder has had on lifestyle and body image.

f. Potential Complications - Bone fragility, infection, death

3. LEUKEMIA

a. Description - A primary malignancy of the bone marrow and lymphatic system which causes overproduction of immature WBCs. The most commonly seen types of leukemia are acute lymphocytic leukemia (80% are ALL) and acute myelogenous (nonlymphocytic) leukemia (AML or ANL). The prognosis of leukemia depends upon staging of the cancer.

    b. **Signs and Symptoms** - Anemia, pallor, fractures, fever, bone pain, fatigue, lassitude, anorexia, frequent infections, bleeding episodes, petechiae, lymphadenopathy, hepatosplenomegaly, hyperuremia

    c. **Diagnostic Procedures** - Diagnosed by history of signs and symptoms, blood smears revealing immature WBC, CBC reveals anemia, neutropenia, thrombocytopenia; bone marrow aspiration and lumbar puncture reveal abnormal cells

    d. **Medical Interventions**

        – **Medications** - Attempt to induce remission by use of chemotherapy according to specific protocol followed by CNS prophylaxis (intrathecal chemotherapy) and maintenance therapy for 30-36 months.

        – **Treatments** - Administer radiation therapy (in some cases).

        – **Surgery -** Bone marrow transplantation may be necessary

    e. **Nursing Interventions** - (See previous list of General Nursing Interventions)

        – **Assessment and Actions**

          • While hospitalized monitor VS, nutritional intake, I & O, bleeding episodes, level of activity tolerance, and level of comfort.

          • Emphasize prevention of infection and prompt treatment of minor injuries (neutropenic precautions, possibly wearing helmet to protect brain, avoidance of dangerous activities such as diving).

          • Discuss life threatening potential of contracting chicken pox and need for prompt treatment if thought to be exposed.

          • Discuss need for platelet transfusion and frequency.

          • Provide antiemetic medication to prevent or diminish nausea.

        – **Teaching**

          • Explain procedures, treatment regimen and side effects of medications.

          • Explain need to prevent injury to any area, utilize soft tooth brush or toothettes.

          • Explain importance of maintaining nutrition and fluid intake.

          • Teach parents signs and symptoms which require MD to be notified (fever, bleeding, pain, extreme fatigue).

        – **Emotional Care**

          • Discuss impact disease has on family and child.

    f. **Potential Complications** - Infections, relapse, death

4. HODGKIN'S LYMPHOMA

    a. **Description** - A malignant growth in the lymphoid system. It often metastasizes to other organs such as the liver, bone marrow, spleen, and lungs. It is treated according to the stage of the neoplasm:

stages 1-5. It affects adolescents more frequently than younger age groups and males more than females. It has a good prognosis.

b. **Signs and Symptoms** - Enlarged, nontender, moveable lymph nodes typically in cervical area; fever, nausea, vomiting, weight loss, cough, night sweats, generalized pruritus, splenomegaly; other symptoms depend upon areas of metastasis

c. **Diagnostic Procedures** - Diagnosed by history and physical, CBC reveals neutrophilia, eosinophilia, lymphocytopenia; bone scan reveals focal or diffuse involvement of bone marrow; biopsy reveals abnormal cells

d. **Medical Interventions**
   - **Medications** - Administer chemotherapy according to specific protocol.
   - **Treatments** - Administer radiation therapy.
   - **Surgery** - May require surgical removal of tumors that have metastasized, may require splenectomy and laparotomy.

e. **Nursing Interventions** - (See previous list of General Nursing Interventions)
   - **Assessment and Actions**
     • Be alert for signs and symptoms.
     • Discuss diagnosis treatment with family.
     • Monitor for side effects of chemotherapy.
     • Preoperatively provide comfort measures and monitor vital signs.
     • Postoperatively monitor vital signs, level of comfort, incision, bowel sounds, and for signs of infection.
     • Be alert to signs indicating potential complications.
   - **Teaching**
     • Instruct family and child on methods to reduce side effects of treatment.
     • Prepare child and family for treatment regimen by describing what to expect before and during and after surgical procedure.
   - **Emotional Care**
     • Discuss how diagnosis and treatment regimen have impacted child's and family's life.

f. **Potential Complications** - Infections, pulmonary emboli from lymphangiography, delayed secondary sexual development, death if widespread metastasis present

5. NEUROBLASTOMAS

- **a. Description** - Tumors which develop from the embryonic neural crest cells. They typically affect the adrenal gland and peritoneal structures. They are classified and treated according to staging (IV-S). They have a poor prognosis.

- **b. Signs and Symptoms** - Usually asymptomatic until after metastasis occurs; symptoms depend on site affected; typically palpable abdominal mass, change in voiding with frequency or retention, lymphadenopathy, periorbital edema and ecchymosis, heterochromia (irises of different colors) if ophthalmic sympathetic nerves involved, cardinal signs of cancer

- **c. Diagnostic Procedures** - Diagnosed by physical findings, CT scan identifies site(s), IV pyelogram determines kidney involvement, clumped cancer cells on bone marrow aspiration, and biopsy reveals abnormal cells

- **d. Medical Interventions**
  - **Medications** - Administer chemotherapy according to specific protocol.
  - **Treatments** - Administer radiation therapy; dialysis is utilized if nephrectomy necessary.
  - **Surgery** - Surgical removal of tumor(s) may be required (stages I-III), nephrectomy performed if kidney involved, bone marrow transplant often attempted

- **e. Nursing interventions** - (See previous list of General Nursing Interventions)
  - **Assessment and Actions**
    - Prevent palpation of mass after diagnosis is made.
    - Preoperatively monitor vital signs and urine output.
    - Postoperatively monitor vital signs, I&O, urine output, and provide method for reducing discomfort.
  - **Teaching**
    - Reinforce critical nature of diagnosis with parents and child if appropriate.
    - Prepare child for dialysis if treatment warrants by explaining what to expect before, during, and after treatment.
  - **Emotional Care**
    - Encourage child to maintain as routine a lifestyle as possible.
    - Provide support to family during grieving period.

- **f. Potential Complications** - Infection, metastasis, death

6. NON-HODGKIN'S LYMPHOMA

a. Description - A rapidly-metastasizing tumor of the lymphoid system. It is often associated with meningeal and mediastinal involvement. It is more commonly seen in boys. Survival rates are 50-80% but treatment is palliative if relapse occurs.

b. Signs and Symptoms - Depend upon sites affected, lymphadenopathy, fatigue, anorexia, weight loss, night sweats, may exhibit signs of leukemia

c. Diagnostic Procedures - Diagnosed by physical findings, biopsy reveals abnormal cells, bone marrow aspiration reveals abnormal cells, x-ray reveals location, and CT scan determines area affected

d. Medical Interventions

   – **Medications** - Administer chemotherapy according to specific protocol.

   – **Treatments** - Administer radiation therapy.

   – **Surgery** - Surgical resection and excision may be performed in some cases.

e. Nursing Interventions - (See previous list of General Nursing Interventions)

   – **Assessment and Actions**

   • Implement nursing care similar to treating the child with leukemia.

   • Monitor patients VS, I & O, nutritional status.

   • Assess level of discomfort and provide means for pain control.

   – **Teaching**

   • Explain diagnosis and treatment plan.

   • Teach importance of meeting nutritional requirements and means for meeting caloric intake.

   • Teach parents about medications prescribed (drug, dose, route, time, and side effects).

   – **Emotional Care**

   • Discuss impact diagnosis has on family and child.

   • Provide support during grieving period.

f. Potential Complications - Infections, death

7. OSTEOGENIC SARCOMA (OSTEOSARCOMA)

a. Description - A malignancy affecting bone tissue (particularly long bones). It is the most commonly seen bone tumor in children. It frequently metastasizes to the lungs and is more common in males and may be related to adolescent growth spurts. It is rare before age 10 and is most common between 10 and 25.

b. Signs and Symptoms - Dull aching or pain in bone, may exhibit limp or guarded extremity, decreased activity level, swelling or redness in area, other cardinal signs of cancer

c. Diagnostic Procedures - Diagnosed by considering history and physical assessment, CT scan reveals location, X-ray reveals sunburst or ray of needles in bone formation, bone scan reveals location and extent of disease

d. Medical Interventions

   – **Medications** - Administer chemotherapy according to specific protocol.

   – **Treatments** - Radiation therapy is ineffective as tumor is radioresistant.

   – **Surgery** - Surgical removal of bone with prosthetic replacement or amputation of extremity is performed.

e. Nursing Interventions - (See previous list of General Nursing Interventions)

   – **Assessment and Actions**

     • Preoperatively provide pain control therapy.

     • Postoperatively monitor vital signs, hemorrhaging status, elevate amputated extremity above the heart, monitor I&O, provide pain control.

     • Provide stump care and be prepared for child to complain of phantom limb pain or sensations.

     • Assist child with ambulation with prosthetic device as soon as possible to promote self mobilization.

   – **Teaching**

     • Discuss amputation and what will happen before, during, and after surgery.

     • Teach stump care to family and application of prosthesis.

     • Teach family and child to protect newly-amputated area and be alert to signs of infection.

     • Reinforce expectations of bone prosthesis (may not be able to walk without crutches, run, swim, or ride a bike).

   – **Emotional Care**

     • Prepare child and family for surgical resection or amputation.

     • Provide support to family during grieving period.

     • Provide time for child and family to discuss change in body image and identify ways that child can cope.

     • Promote normal growth and development throughout treatment.

f. Potential Complications - Infection, lung metastasis, death

8. RETINOBLASTOMA

a. Description - A hereditary neoplastic tumor of the retina. It arises from transmission of a mutated, defective gene or spontaneous cell mutations. The prognosis depends upon the staging (Group 1-best prognosis, Group 5 poor prognosis). The symptoms usually occur before two years of age. Survival rate is good but may include loss of vision.

b. Signs and Symptoms - White reflex in eye (appears as Cat's eye reflex on simple visual inspection) often accompanied by strabismus and change in visual acuity; may cause blindness in late stage

c. Diagnostic Procedures - Diagnosed by abnormal findings in ophthalmic examination during scleral indentation, fiberoptic transillumination, and tomograms of orbit; also presence of elevated LDH in aqueous humor

d. Medical Interventions

  – **Medications** - Administer chemotherapy.

  – **Treatments** - Depends upon staging; staging 1-3 require radiation therapy; photocoagulation, cryotherapy, or radioactive applicators may be utilized

  – **Surgery** - States 1-3 require cryotherapy and coagulation of specific retinal blood vessels; stages 4-5 often require surgical enucleation.

e. Nursing Interventions - (See previous list of General Nursing Interventions)

  – **Assessment and Actions**

  • Assess vision before and after treatment.

  • Monitor for signs of infection postoperatively.

  • Provide method of pain control.

  – **Teaching**

  • Teach parents care of and placement of prosthetic device and orbital socket.

  • Assist parent and child in maintaining a safe environment and help child adapt to visual change and, if appropriate, loss of eye.

  – **Emotional Care**

  • Prepare child and family for appearance after enucleation.

  • Discuss impact on family and how family is coping.

f. Potential Complications - Blindness, infection

9. RHABDOMYOSARCOMA

a. Description - A malignant tumor of the soft tissue (muscles, connective tissue, lymphatic tissue, tendons, vascular tissue). It arises from embryonal tissue and may occur anywhere in the body where striated muscle is found. It occurs most often between 2 and 6 years and 15 and 19 years. It is staged according to the sites and metastasis (Group 1-4). Forty percent occur in the head, orbit and neck, 35% in genitourinary and abdominal areas and 25% in the trunk and extremities. The prognosis is good if remission is achieved. If relapse occurs survival rate is poor.

   b. Signs and Symptoms - Depends upon site of tumor but most common signs are painless mass or functional impairment of affected site; may also include: visible mass, wound which does not heal, pain in area, swelling, frequent ear infections, lymphadenopathy; symptoms may not occur until tumor becomes enlarged and begins to put pressure on other tissues in the area

   c. Diagnostic Procedures - Diagnosed by direct inspection and palpation, X-ray and CT scans reveal location, bone marrow aspiration and lumbar puncture show abnormal cells, MRI shows location and size of tumor; tissue biopsy reveals abnormal cells

   d. Medical Interventions
   - **Medications** - Administer chemotherapy according to specific protocol.
   - **Treatments** - Administer radiation therapy.
   - **Surgery** - Surgical removal of tumor performed if tumor can be completely excised.

   e. Nursing Interventions - (See previous list of General Nursing Interventions)
   - **Assessment and Actions**
     • Provide method for pain control.
     • Assess for signs of infection and treat promptly.
   - **Teaching**
     • Explain prognosis and provide emotional support to family and child.
   - **Emotional Care**
     • Promote normal growth and development for child.
     • Discuss impact diagnosis has on child and family.

   f. Potential Complications - Infection, death

10. WILM'S TUMOR (NEPHROBLASTOMA)

   a. Description - A malignant, encapsulated tumor located in the kidney. It may also be accompanied by other congenital anomalies (genitourinary anomalies, aniridia). It usually affects the left kidney. It arises from embryonic tissue and is most often seen between 1 and 5 years, with peak incidence between 3 and 4 years of age. It is staged from 1-5 according to the growth and level of metastasis. It has a good prognosis especially for Stages 1-3.

b. **Signs and Symptoms** - Abdominal mass palpable (firm, nontender), increase in abdominal girth, hematuria, hypertension (25% of cases), and anemia

c. **Diagnostic Procedures** - Diagnosed by IV pyelogram, abdominal CT scan, presence of polycythemia, and urinalysis

d. **Medical Interventions**

  – **Medications** - Administer chemotherapy according to specific protocols.

  – **Treatments** - Administer radiation therapy.

  – **Surgery** - Surgical removal of the kidney, adrenal gland and tumorous mass; other tissue which may be affected (lymph nodes) is also removed during this surgical procedure

e. **Nursing Interventions** - (See previous list of General Nursing Interventions)

  – **Assessment and Actions**

  • Avoid further palpation of the tumor before surgery.

  • Provide postoperative care to child providing for comfort.

  – **Teaching**

  • Prepare family and child for surgery (usually within 24-48 hours after detection of tumor).

  • Prepare child and family for side effects of treatment regimen.

  • Instruct family and child on importance of maintaining complete function of the remaining kidney, report signs of UTI or kidney infection promptly.

  – **Emotional Care**

  • Discuss impact diagnosis and treatment regimen have on family and child's life.

f. **Potential Complications** - Infection, paralytic ileus (postoperatively), kidney failure or infection.

13

HEMATOLOGICAL DISORDERS

I. General Concepts

- Blood is primarily formed from the bone marrow. It is composed of:

  - **Plasma** - water (90%) and proteins, electrolytes, glucose, fats, fibrinogen (10%)
  - **Cells** - erythrocytes, leukocytes, and platelets

- Blood functions to bring oxygen to the tissues; buffer the fluid and electrolytes; repair injuries or infections, transport nutrients and waste products, and regulate the body's temperature.

II. Specific Hematology Disorders

Congenital

1. COOLEY'S ANEMIA (BETA-THALASSEMIA MAJOR)

   a. Description - An autosomal co-dominant genetic trait in which there is diminished production of the beta globin chain of hemoglobin A causing severe anemia. It is primarily seen among the Black, Oriental and Mediterranean population. Typically the symptoms develop after six months of life. The child's bone marrow is hyperplastic and the RBCs are fragile. They seldom live until adulthood.

   b. Signs and Symptoms - Severe anemia, splenomegaly, headache, anorexia, weakness, pallor, bone pain, flat bones of face characteristically widened, hemosiderosis, bronze skin appearance, fibrosis of major organs, (gallbladder, heart, liver, pancreas, spleen), delayed physical growth and sexual maturation

   c. Diagnostic Procedures - Diagnosed by CBC revealing anemia, hemoglobin electrophoresis shows elevated reticulocyte count, elevated bilirubin; X-ray shows increased medullary area with thinning of cortex

d. Medical Interventions

   – **Medications** - Administer folic acid and testosterone; administer prophylactic antibiotic therapy postoperatively.

   – **Treatments** - Administer blood transfusions (packed red blood cells), perform chelation.

   – **Surgery** - Splenectomy may be necessary

e. Nursing Interventions

   – **Assessment and Actions**
   - Be alert to signs and symptoms indicating disorder.
   - Assess child before during and after transfusion (vital signs and signs of transfusion reactions).
   - Refer parents to genetic counseling.
   - Assess for signs indicating potential complications.

   – **Teaching**
   - Explain diagnosis to parents and child and discuss treatment regimen.
   - Discuss with parents the need for frequent transfusions.

   – **Emotional Care**
   - Provide support to family and child.
   - Support and facilitate grieving process.

   f. Potential Complications - Heart failure, diabetes, cirrhosis of the liver, cholelithiasis, hemosiderosis, death

2. HEMOPHILIA (CLASSIC)

a. Description - A bleeding disorder, typically occurring in males, that is due to a deficiency in one of the normal clotting factors. The most common type (75%) is Hemophilia A in which Factor VIII is deficient. The severity of the disease ranges from mild to severe bleeding tendencies.

b. Signs and Symptoms - Depend upon severity; frequent bruising or bleeding which is difficult to stop; hemarthrosis, epistaxis, internal and/or spontaneous hemorrhaging, joint pain and stiffness, hematuria

c. Diagnostic Procedures - Diagnosed by presence of abnormalities in blood clotting tests (PT, PTT, TGT, fibrinogen level) and absence or deficiency in Factor VIII

d. Medical Interventions

- **Medications** - Administer corticosteroids to reduce inflammation of hemarthrosis.
- **Treatments** - Administer (IV) missing Factor VIII; physical therapy to prevent loss of joint mobility.
- **Surgery** - Unnecessary

e. Nursing Interventions

- **Assessment and Actions**
  - Be alert to signs and symptoms.
  - Obtain thorough history considering past bleeding episodes.
  - Refer parents to genetic counseling.
  - Monitor child's vital signs, and for reaction during transfusion.
  - Assess for signs indicating potential complications.

- **Teaching**
  - Explain diagnosis to parents and child and discuss treatment regimen.
  - Explain administration of Factor VIII including frequency, duration and side effects.
  - Explain how to prevent and control bleeding such as discouraging contact sports, utilizing soft tooth brush, maintaining normal weight for age to prevent further joint abuse, applying pressure to any cuts for 10 to 15 minutes as well as applying ice to area, immobilizing joints when swollen, and providing physical therapy once swelling reduced to maintain joint ROM.
  - Teach methods for reducing discomfort (positioning, analgesics, application of cold or warmth).

- **Emotional Care**
  - Determine how parents and child are coping.
  - Encourage child to discuss how disorder affects his life.
  - Provide support to the family and child.
  - Provide support group information to family.

f. Potential Complications - Joint limitations, internal hemorrhaging, transfusion reactions, increased potential for contracting hepatitis B or AIDS, shock, and death

3. **HYPERBILIRUBINEMIA IN THE NEWBORN (NEWBORN JAUNDICE)**

   a. **Description** - An overabundance of bilirubin in the blood stream. It often occurs in neonates (icterus neonatorum) and may be due to the immaturity of the liver or be due to Rh incompatibility (erythroblastosis fetalis)

   b. **Signs and Symptoms** - Jaundice, elevated total bilirubin levels greater than 12 mg/dl

   c. **Diagnostic Procedures** - Diagnosed by assessing direct and indirect bilirubin levels, maternal blood group and Rh typing, and presence of positive direct and indirect Coomb's test

   d. **Medical Interventions**
   - **Medications** - Administer RhoGAM to mothers who are Rh negative to prevent this problems with successive births
   - **Treatments** - Administer phototherapy, monitor bilirubin levels, and possibly administer exchange transfusions (prn)
   - **Surgery** - Unnecessary

   e. **Nursing Interventions**
   - **Assessment and Actions**
     - Assess newborn for jaundice by inspecting sclera and skin.
     - If phototherapy used: cover infants eyes and genitals in male; remove eye shields every feeding and when not under the lights; turn nude infant every 2 hours to expose all surface areas to light; maintain infant's temperature
     - Maintain hydration status of infant during therapy (frequent feedings and/or IV therapy).
     - Monitor bilirubin levels as ordered.
     - If exchange transfusion utilized, monitor infant's vital signs, amount of blood removed and transfused, and for signs of reaction.
     - Assess for signs of CNS changes (kernicterus) until level within normal range.
   - **Teaching**
     - Explain diagnosis to parents and discuss treatment regimen.
     - If home therapy utilized, instruct parents in care.
   - **Emotional Care**
     - Encourage parents to care for and interact with child.
     - Provide support and allow parents to ask questions.

   f. **Potential Complications** - Kernicterus/brain damage

4. SICKLE CELL ANEMIA

a. Description - An autosomal disorder in which an erythrocyte containing Hemoglobin S (Hb S) becomes sickled in shape when decreased oxygen is present. The sickled erythrocyte either hemolyzes or causes sluggish blood flow, thus decreasing its ability to carry oxygen. This disorder is usually found in the Black population but may also be present in individuals from the Arabian Peninsula, Greece, Turkey and India. Sickle cell anemia may be life-threatening if a severe crisis occurs. Sickle cell trait is defined as those individuals who have less than 50% of HbS. People with sickle cell trait are typically asymptomatic unless under external stressors (vigorous exercise, illness, exposure to high altitudes) where oxygenation is diminished.

b. Signs and Symptoms - (Sickle Cell Crisis) Complaint of pain in joint, back or abdomen, hand-foot syndrome (pain and swelling in hands and feet); poor wound healing; decreased growth; enlargement of spleen and liver; osteoporosis; priapism; hematuria; pale mucous membranes; ischemia may cause CVA and kidney malfunction

c. Diagnostic Procedures - Diagnosed by presence of sickled RBC on blood smears, positive Sickledex, and evidence of sickling with hemoglobin electrophoresis

d. Medical Interventions

- **Medications** - Administer antibiotic for infection (if present), analgesics during sickle cell crisis.
- **Treatments** - Provide for adequate oxygenation, rest, hydration, and pain control measures; blood transfusions may be necessary.
- **Surgery** - Splenectomy may be necessary.

e. Nursing Interventions

- **Assessment and Actions**
  - Be alert to signs and symptoms.
  - Refer parents to genetic counseling.
  - During crisis promote oxygenation, hydration, bedrest.
  - Provide method for reducing discomfort (warm compresses to area, elevating extremity).

- **Teaching**
  - Explain diagnosis to parents and child and discuss treatment regimen.
  - Teach parents and child how to prevent sickle cell crisis, treat infections promptly, maintain hydration status, avoid exercise that causes rapid oxygen depletion, diminish stressors.

- **Emotional Care**
  - Discuss chronicity of disease and how family is coping.
  - Provide support to family and child.
  - Provide information regarding support group.

f. **Potential Complications** - CVA, blindness, cirrhosis of the liver, chronic ulceration of lower extremities, hepatomegaly, splenomegaly, heart failure, death.

Acquired

1. IDIOPATHIC THROMBOCYTOPENIC PURPURA (ITP)

a. **Description** - An acute or chronic condition in which there is excessive damage and destruction of the platelets in the spleen. It is an autoimmune disorder. The acute form often follows an upper respiratory infection or communicable disease (rubella, varicella, or rubeola). Most children recover spontaneously.

b. **Signs and Symptoms** - Ecchymosis with petechiae, hematuria, hematemesis, bleeding gums, ecchymosis on lower extremities, epistaxis

c. **Diagnostic Procedures** - Diagnosed by platelet count being <20,000/mm^3/dL; tourniquet test reveals petechiae formation and bone marrow aspiration reveals reduced number of platelets

d. **Medical Interventions**
   - **Medications** - Administer corticosteroids, gamma globulin.
   - **Treatments** - Provide supportive care and safety since disorder is self-limiting; may require platelet transfusion if hemorrhaging occurs.
   - **Surgery** - Usually unnecessary; splenectomy may be required

e. **Nursing Interventions**
   *See previous interventions for Hemophilia

   - **Assessment and Actions**
     • Be alert to signs and symptoms indicating disorder.
     • Obtain thorough history to determine cause.
     • Monitor for signs and symptoms of transfusion reaction.
   - **Teaching**
     • Explain diagnosis to parents and discuss treatment regimen.
     • Teach ways to prevent further bleeding episodes: omit contact sports or physical activity, maintain weight within normal limits, limit heavy lifting and stress to joints, utilize soft toothbrush, reduce chance for infection
     • Explain need for transfusion (prn).
   - **Emotional Care**
     • Provide parents and child time to ask questions and voice concerns.
     • Provide support to family and child.

f. **Potential Complications** - Transfusion reaction, hemorrhaging, shock, death if severe

2. IRON-DEFICIENCY ANEMIA

a. **Description** - A type of anemia which may be due to inadequate intake of iron (most common), increased iron needs, diminished iron stores, blood loss, or malabsorption. It is most commonly seen in infancy due to an over-consumption of milk and an iron-poor diet. It is most frequently seen in infants from 6 months to 3 years of age.

b. **Signs and Symptoms** - Usually exhibits a gradual onset of signs and symptoms; fat baby or child, edema, limited activity level, fatigue, porcelain-like skin, paleness, muscle weakness, tachycardia, petechiae

c. **Diagnostic Procedures** - Diagnosed by CBC which reveals hypochromic microcytic RBC, decreased hemoglobin, elevated RBC, decreased reticulocyte count, decreased serum iron concentration, and stool testing (positive guaiac may be present if due to hemorrhaging)

d. **Medical Interventions**

  - **Medications** - Administer oral ferrous sulfate or IV iron dextran, administer ascorbic acid with iron to enhance GI absorption.

  - **Treatments** - Increase iron in diet, correcting underlying causes, and administer blood transfusion if severe anemia present.

  - **Surgery** - Unnecessary

e. **Nursing Interventions**

  - **Assessment and Actions**
    - Be alert to signs and symptoms.
    - Obtain thorough history to determine cause.
    - Encourage rest periods and slowly increase activity level once child has begun treatment.
    - Make parents aware that periodic screening may be done to assess child's progress.
    - Assess for signs indicating potential complications.

  - **Teaching**
    - Prevent occurrence by encouraging iron supplements in infancy and including dark green leafy vegetables, red meats, organ meats or whole grains in child's diet.
    - Explain diagnosis to family and discuss treatment regimen.
    - Teach parents proper method of administering iron supplements: administer at back of mouth to prevent tooth staining, brush teeth after administration, administer with orange juice to enhance absorption.
    - Warn parents stools may become darker with oral iron administration and child may become constipated; prevent constipation by exercising, high fiber diet, and increasing fluids.
    - Instruct parents to decrease child's milk intake and provide other foods.

  - **Emotional Care**

- Provide support to family and child.

f. **Potential Complications** - Growth failure or delay, heart failure

14

IMMUNE DISORDERS

I. General Concepts

- The immune system is composed of primary organs (thymus and bone marrow) and secondary organs (tonsils, adenoids, lymph nodes, and spleen).

- The immune system functions to protect the body against disease.

- The immune system provides specific and nonspecific immunity.

    * Specific immunity includes the reactions of the body to specific recognized foreign bodies and is composed of cell-mediated and humoral defense mechanisms.

    1. Cell-mediated response: T-lymphocyte mediated response
    2. Humoral mediated response: complement, B-lymphocytes and plasma cells (IgA, IgD, IgE, IgM, IgG) mediated response

    * Nonspecific immunity includes the body's ability to react to any foreign body regardless of previous exposure (primarily the process of phagocytosis and inflammation).

- Immunity may be actively or passively-acquired and be a natural or artificial immunity (details in the Communicable Disease section).

- Immunological disorders may be due to a defect of the stem cell, T-cell, B-cell, or phagocyte.

- The immune system may be affected by alterations in genetic make-up, nutrition, metabolism, anatomy or environmental factors.

II. Specific Immune Disorders

Congenital Disorders

1. SEVERE COMBINED IMMUNODEFICIENCY SYNDROME (SCID)

a. **Description** - An inherited disorder in which cellular and humoral immunity are absent. It has a poor prognosis.

b. **Signs and Symptoms** - increased susceptibility to infection after 3 months of age, vomiting, cough, *Candida* diaper rash, recurrence of infections or infections without complete recovery, FTT, diarrhea, thrush

c. **Diagnostic Procedures** - Diagnosed by considering history of frequent and recurrent infections, and assessing blood for lymphocytopenia, presence of decreased plasma cells in bone marrow, and body's inability to respond to antigens

d. **Medical Interventions**
   - **Medications** - Administer immunoglobulin.
   - **Treatments** - Keep child in sterile environment (Bubble boy).
   - **Surgery** - Bone marrow transplant may be recommended.

e. **Nursing Interventions**
   - **Assessment and Actions**
     - Be alert for signs and symptoms indicating disorder.
     - Provide child with sterile environment.
     - Prevent and treat infections promptly.
     - Refer parents to genetic counseling.
     - If bone marrow transplant attempted, provide sterile environment and monitor child for signs of graft vs. host reaction (febrile episodes, diarrhea, hepatosplenomegaly, skin eruptions)
     - Assess for signs indicating potential complications.
   - **Teaching**
     - Assess parents' and child's understanding of disease.
     - Discuss ways to minimize infections (handwashing, maintaining thorough hygiene, prevent exposing child to others who are ill).
   - **Emotional Care**
     - Promote normal growth and development for age (see unit on Growth and Development).
     - Encourage child to discuss feelings.
     - Determine family's level of coping and offer suggestions on ways to cope with situation.

- Provide support to family and child.

f. Potential Complications - Graft vs. host reactio, which is irreversible, death from infection or transplant rejection

Acquired Disorders

1. ACQUIRED IMMUNODEFICIENCY SYNDROME

a. Description - This disorder is commonly referred to as AIDS, HIV, or HTLV 3. It is a fatal disorder in which the body becomes infected by the Human T-cell Lymphotrophic virus. Once infected, the body is unable to fight off opportunistic infections. The virus is transferred via the placenta, blood, IV drug abuse, semen, and, possibly, vaginal secretions . The majority of children affected with this virus are under the age of two (77% infected prenatally).

b. Signs and Symptoms - FTT, vomiting, diarrhea, frequent and recurrent oral monilial infections, lymphadenopathy, pneumonitis, hepatosplenomegaly, microcephaly (in some cases)

c. Diagnostic Procedures - Diagnosed by ruling out other possible immune disorders; noting presence of opportunistic infections, positive antibody to HTLV 3, positive HIV in blood

d. Medical Interventions

- **Medications** - Administer Zidovudine (AZT), gamma globulin, antibiotics for infections.
- **Treatments** - Provide supportive care, managing infections promptly; there is no cure.
- **Surgery** - Unnecessary

e. Nursing Interventions

- **Assessment and Actions**
  - Be alert to signs and symptoms of disorder.
  - Determine mode of transmission and if others in family are HIV positive.
  - Utilize Universal Precautions and encourage thorough handwashing when in contact with child.
  - Encourage well-balanced nutritional intake.
  - Prevent child from being exposed to possible infections.
  - Refer parents and child for counseling.
- **Teaching**
  - Explain diagnosis to parents and child (if appropriate for age).
  - Instruct on mode of transmission and encourage social interaction with child by family and peers.
  - Teach parents about medication prescribed (drug, dose, route, side effects).
- **Emotional Care**
  - Encourage expression of feelings.

- Promote child's development and growth.
- Enhance self-esteem and quality of child's life.
- Attempt to maintain routines in child's life.
- Promote positive family communication.
- Provide support to family and child.
- Provide support group information to family.

f. Potential Complications - Pneumonia, other opportunistic infections, skin lesions, often social isolation, and death

2. ANAPHYLAXIS

a. Description - A hypersensitivity reaction in response to an allergen to which the child has been previously exposed.

b. Signs and Symptoms - Rapid reaction of all body systems (usually occurs within seconds or minutes after exposure), rhinitis, nausea, vomiting, flushing, tachycardia, hypotension, urticaria, wheezing, bronchospasm, seizures, loss of consciousness, syncope; symptoms may vary in severity

c. Diagnostic Procedures - Diagnosed by rapid onset of symptoms, physical findings and history

d. Medical Interventions

- **Medications** - Depend upon severity but may include administration of diphenhydramine (mild reaction), epinephrine or aminophylline administration
- **Treatments** - Provide supportive care (oxygen, airway maintenance, IV fluids) for a patient in shock; ventilation may be necessary.
- **Surgery** - Unnecessary

e. Nursing Interventions

- **Assessment and Actions**
  - Be alert to signs and symptoms as prompt detection may be life-saving for child.
  - Monitor vital signs, respiratory status, neurological status, and I&O.
  - Assist with administration of medication as ordered.
  - Identify allergy exposed to and instruct parents and child to attempt to prevent further exposure, if possible.
  - Encourage child to wear a Medic Alert bracelet or tag.
  - Alert teachers, school nurse, and friends of possible allergen, signs of reactions and treatment regimen.
- **Teaching**
  - Explain diagnosis to parents and child and discuss treatment regimen.
  - Teach parents how to recognize future reactions and treat by carrying and using diphenhydramine or epinephrine injector.

   – **Emotional Care**
- Provide support to family and child.

f. Potential Complications - Death if untreated

APPENDIX A

Growth Charts

Girls: Birth to 36 Months
Physical Growth NCHS Percentiles*

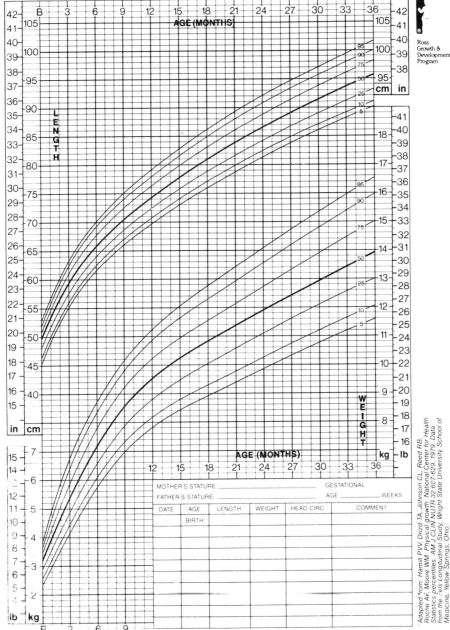

Girls: Birth to 36 Months
Physical Growth NCHS Percentiles*

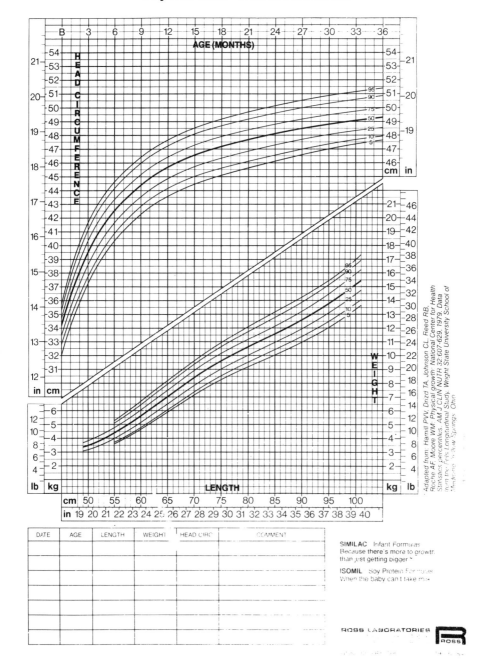

DATE	AGE	LENGTH	WEIGHT	HEAD CIRC	COMMENT

SIMILAC Infant Formulas
Because there's more to growth
than just getting bigger.*

ISOMIL Soy Protein Formulas
When the baby can't take milk

Adapted from: Hamill PVV, Drizd TA, Johnson CL, Reed RB,
Roche AF, Moore WM. Physical growth: National Center for Health
Statistics percentiles. AM J CLIN NUTR 32:607-629, 1979. Data
from the Fels Longitudinal Study, Wright State University School of
Medicine, Yellow Springs, Ohio.

ROSS LABORATORIES

Girls: Prepubescent
Physical Growth NCHS Percentiles*

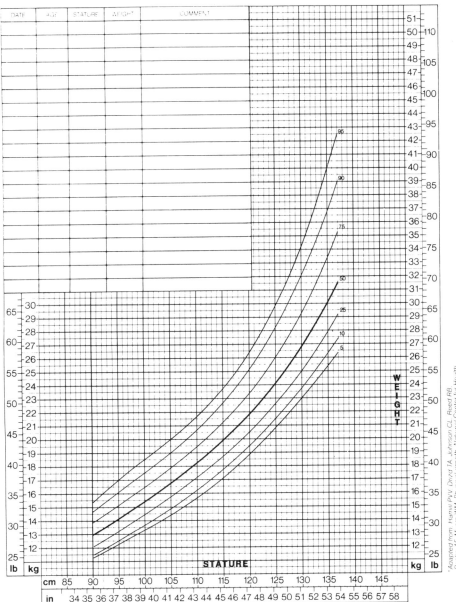

SIMILAC® Infant Formulas
First choice of more physicians
and used in more hospitals

ISOMIL® Soy Protein Formulas
First choice of more physicians
for milk-free feeding

ROSS LABORATORIES
COLUMBUS OHIO 43216

51214 09893WB
(0 05) NOVEMBER 1991   LITHO IN USA

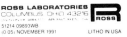

Girls: 2 to 18 Years
Physical Growth NCHS Percentiles*

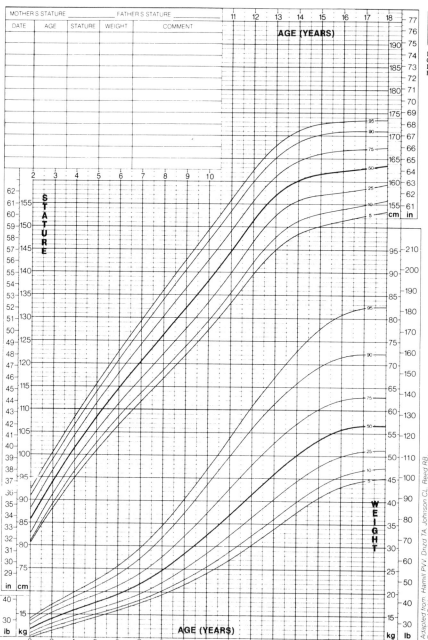

Boys: Birth to 36 Months
Physical Growth NCHS Percentiles*

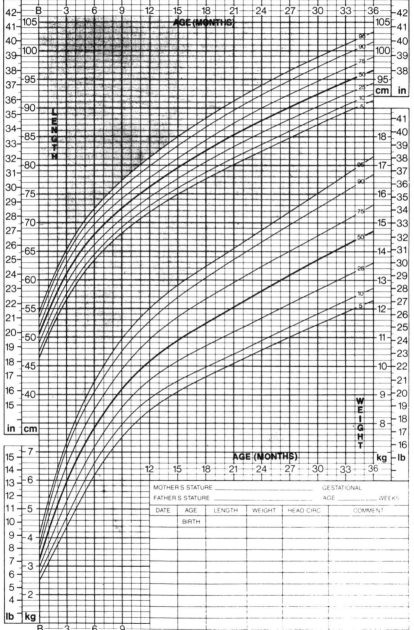

Ross
Growth &
Development
Program

Adapted from: Hamil PVV, Drizd TA, Johnson CL, Reed RB, Roche AF, Moore WM. Physical growth: National Center for Health Statistics percentiles. AM J CLIN NUTR 32:607-629, 1979. Data from the Fels Longitudinal Study, Wright State University School of Medicine, Yellow Springs, Ohio

MOTHER'S STATURE _____   GESTATIONAL
FATHER'S STATURE _____   AGE _____ WEEKS

DATE	AGE	LENGTH	WEIGHT	HEAD CIRC	COMMENT
	BIRTH				

Boys: Birth to 36 Months
Physical Growth NCHS Percentiles*

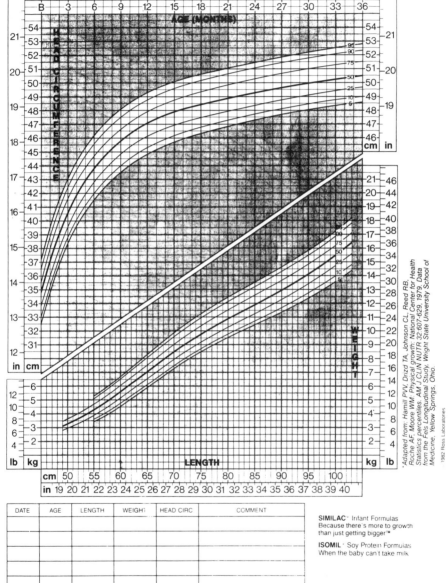

DATE	AGE	LENGTH	WEIGHT	HEAD CIRC	COMMENT

SIMILAC Infant Formulas
Because there's more to growth
than just getting bigger™

ISOMIL Soy Protein Formulas
When the baby can't take milk

Boys: Prepubescent
Physical Growth NCHS Percentiles*

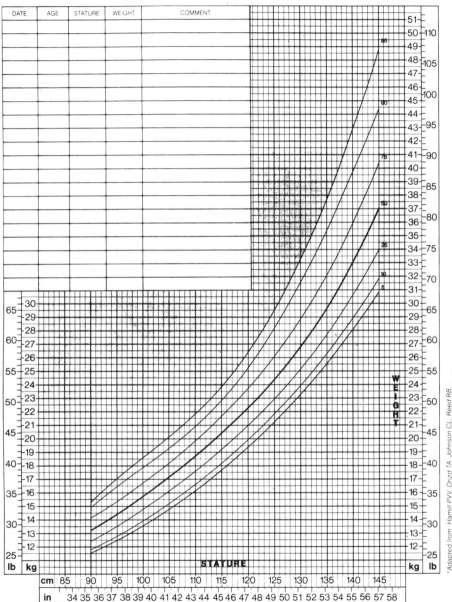

DATE	AGE	STATURE	WEIGHT	COMMENT

Boys: 2 to 18 Years
Physical Growth NCHS Percentiles*

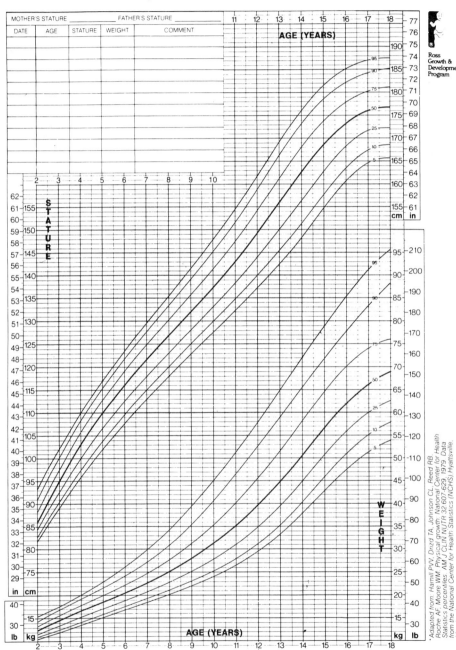

Ross
Growth &
Development
Program

*Adapted from: Hamill PVV, Drizd TA, Johnson CL, Reed RB, Roche AF, Moore WM. Physical growth: National Center for Health Statistics percentiles. AM J CLIN NUTR 32:607-629, 1979. Data from the National Center for Health Statistics (NCHS), Hyattsville, Maryland.

© 1982 Ross Laboratories

APPENDIX B

Growth and Development Assessment
By Brenda Goodner, RN, MSN, CS

This growth and development chart is an assessment of major developmental milestones at a specific age. This is essential information for anyone who assesses children.

BIRTH - 4 MONTHS
- Startle response to noise
- Turns head to direction of voice
- Smiles at another
- Undifferentiated crying
- Grasps at objects when placed in hand
- Holds head up momentarily (4 weeks)
- Begins to hold head constantly (16 weeks)
- Will follow toy within line of sight
- Laughs out loud (16 weeks)
- Stares at own hands
- Looks at himself in mirror

4-6 MONTHS
- Recognizes familiar sounds, recognizes voices
- Reaches for objects, but often misjudges distance
- Full control of head movements
- Enjoys playing with toys
- Sits in highchair
- Rolls from prone to supine
- Pulls up to sit
- Plays bo-peep
- Begins to differentiate likes and dislikes of food

6-9 MONTHS
- Drinks from cup
- Eating solid foods
- Responds to name
- Responds to gestures (bye-bye, pat-a-cake)
- Puts things in mouth
- Says "da" and "bye"
- Feeds self cookie

- May imitate adults
- Rolls from supine to prone
- Becomes fretful when mother leaves

9-12 MONTHS

- Imitates voice sounds
- Speaks first real words
- Offers head and foot while dressing
- Creeps
- Comprehends meaning of mama, dada, bye, no
- Rolls ball to another person

12-15 MONTHS

- Enjoys rhymes
- Identifies objects
- Responds to simple commands
- Begins to recognize wet diaper
- Kisses upon request
- Developing a memory
- May exhibit shyness
- Jabbers in non-meaningful sentences
- Walks with assistance (13 months)
- Drinks from cup, feeds self
- Takes off shoes
- Points at things he wants
- Babinski's reflex

15-18 MONTHS

- Walks without assistance
- Understands simple instructions
- Uses "no" indiscriminantly
- Gains spinchter control
- Expresses emotions, temper tantrums
- Kisses and hugs

18-24 MONTHS

- Listens to simple stories
- Vocabulary increases to 300 words
- Produces word combinations
- Refers to himself by name
- Runs and falls

- Throws ball without falling
- Begins to scribble
- Points to nose, hair
- Asks for food, drinks
- Washes hands
- Builds tower of blocks
- Turns pages of book
- Puts on clothes, shoes
- Talks constantly
- Parallel play (watches others play but does not play with them)

24-30 MONTHS
- Talks in phases
- Turns doorknob
- Takes off lids
- Begins to draw
- Knows first and last name
- Talks constantly
- Has imaginary playmate
- Attention span increasing
- Dresses self

3 YEARS
- Rapid expansion of vocabulary (900 words)
- Identifies objects and what they are for
- Carries on conversation
- Uses simple sentences
- Night-time bladder control
- Learns to ride tricycle
- Asks questions constantly
- Expresses fear of dark
- Realizes own sex
- Parallel and associative play

4 YEARS
- Vocabulary extends to 1500 words
- Fewer grammatical errors
- Exaggerates stories
- Constantly questioning
- Becoming independent
- Strongly attached to parent of opposite sex

- Associative and cooperative play

5 YEARS

- Vocabulary of 2,000 words
- Can count up to ten
- Knows his age
- Knows primary colors
- Sentences more complex
- Aware of handedness
- Ties shoelaces
- Names money
- Can follow 3 instructions at a time
- Eager to please
- Identifies with parent of same sex
- Cooperative play

6 YEARS

- Sentences grammatically correct
- Reads simple stories
- Tends to giggle over nothing
- Aware of days and seasons
- Gaining more independence
- Imitates adults more

APPENDIX C

Health Assessment Tips

Environment
- Quiet, private area
- Temperature of comfort for client
- No bright lights or glare from sun
- Provide comfort, security for client, toddlers; infants on mother's lap; preschooler, schoolage-mother at side; adolescent-determine whether prefers parents presence

Introduction
- Address child and parent; use child's name frequently
- Explain reason for interview, what will happen
- Establish rapport with child using gentle touch, eye contact, speaking to child at eye level
- Assure that information will be kept confidential
- Postpone interview if client is in pain or agitated
- Be attentive and avoid interruptions

Age-related Techniques
- Obtain most of information from parent or reliable source (child's memory is often inaccurate)
- Repeat statements and questions if necessary, allow time to respond
- Incorporate children over 2 years in simple questions to give a sense of control
- Allow for frequent questions; explain in simple terms

APPENDIX D

Health Assessment

Patient's name

Age

Date of birth

Sex

Information

Reliable source

Chief complaint

Onset, location, quality and quantity of discomfort, aggravating and alleviating factors, how has complaint impacted child's life/activity level; treatments (including medications) and response to treatment

Past History

Prenatal

Mother and fetus health status

Complications during pregnancy

Mother's emotional status during pregnancy

Medications prescribed during pregnancy

Birth History

Type of delivery

Complications, if any

Weight, length, APGAR score, gestational age, complications or abnormalities of infant

Growth and Development

Age at which milestones achieved (gross motor, fine motor, cognitive, social ability)

Family Profile

Names and ages of each member of the family

Health status of each family member

Age of onset of illnesses in family

Family interaction

Family support systems

Cultural background

Utilization of health care system

History of child's illnesses

Communicable diseases

Frequency of infections

Immunizations
Accidents
Allergies: food, drug, environment
Current medications
Hospitalizations
Surgeries

Nutrition

Special diet, appetite, vitamin supplement, weight gain or loss

24-Hour History

Review daily activity for child

Review of Systems

Overall appearance

Skin

Color, temperature, masses, diaphoresis, lesions, rashes, dryness, bleeding, edema, scars

Head

Headaches, any evidence of trauma, fontanelles, masses

Eyes

Visual acuity, pruritis, color vision, strabismus, infections, corrective devices used

Ears

Infections, hearing perception, speech

Nose

Drainage, flaring, dyspnea, epistaxis

Mouth and Throat

Infection, number and color of teeth and cavities, tonsils, discomfort

Neck

Enlarged nodes or masses, stiffness, symmetry, ROM

Respiratory

Infections, dyspnea, cough, fever breath sounds (esp. wheezing, rhonchi, crackles, stridor) hoarseness, number of colds per year, hemoptysis

Cardiovascular

Pallor, pulses, cyanosis, fainting episodes, hypertension, known cardiac defects, ability to continue activity, fatigue during exertion, murmurs

Gastrointestinal

Appetite, bowel problems and habits, nausea, vomiting, cramping, diarrhea, constipation, flatulence, abdominal symmetry, bowel sounds, abdominal rigidity

Genitourinary

Frequency, odor, dysuria, hematuria, polyuria, incontinence, discharge, infections

Musculoskeletal

Discomfort, edema, ROM, gait, injuries, strength, posture, symmetry, color, temperature, fracture, deformities, scoliosis

Neurological

Headaches, seizures, syncope, dizziness, coordination, unusual behavior, change in level of consciousness, reflexes appropriate to age

Endocrine

Growth pattern, adjustments to climate, excessive thirst, diaphoresis, presence of sexual characteristics

Reproductive

Male: Descended testes, Tanner stage: development of secondary sex characteristics; masses, infection

Female: Onset of menses, regularity of menses, Tanner stage: development of secondary sex characteristics; masses, infection

APPENDIX E

Physical Assessment

Environment

- Provide well-lighted setting
- Decrease noise and distractions
- Ensure safety for infant, child/parent
- Provide for privacy
- Properly drape for privacy, utilize extra blanket for warmth
- Warm hands and instruments before touching client
- Place client in sitting or supine position depending on system being examined
- Allow to empty bladder before examination

Procedures for Examination

Infants and Toddlers

- Introduce self
- Allow parent or caretaker to hold infant or child when possible
- Utilize a slow approach and establish rapport with child and parent
- Allow parent to assist with positioning when necessary to allow a sense of control
- Obtain "quiet" vital signs and assessment items that require auscultation first (respirations and lung fields, apical pulse, heart sounds, and abdominal sounds)
- Remember that obtaining blood pressure and temperature may cause discomfort. This may be done after need for silence is over
- Utilize play and interact with client to maintain rapport
- Examine eyes, ears, nose, throat last
- Talk with parent or caretaker in a soft, gentle voice throughout exam explaining each area being assessed
- Maintain normal temperature throughout exam by keeping infant/toddler in a blanket or sheet and assessing one area at a time
- Answer all questions and concerns, inform of use of information
- Inform if any further examination needed
- Discuss findings with parent
- Provide educational information to parent, prn

Preschooler

- Introduce self, establish rapport
- Explain each portion of exam in simple terms before performing

- Place child in a position near parent that is safe
- Assess the child interacting at eye level
- Approach slowly, examine in a toe-to-head direction leaving eyes, ears, nose, throat for last
- Assess "quiet" vital signs and areas first (respirations and lung fields, apical pulse, heart sounds, and abdominal sounds) before invasive procedures are assessed
- Describe to child what blood pressure will feel like to reduce surprise effect
- Describe to child how they may assist with exam
- Have parent assist with undressing child; provide a drape for privacy
- Allow preschooler to examine equipment prior to use, to alleviate anxiety
- Stress normal findings throughout exam
- Apply a bandaid over invasive procedures which injure the skin
- Discuss findings with parent
- Provide educational information to parent prn
- Answer all questions and concerns, inform if any further examination needed

School-Age
- Introduce self
- Establish rapport
- Explain procedures to child/parent
- Describe length of time exam will take and child's role
- Position child safely on exam table or bed with parent in room
- Ask if child has any questions before beginning exam, during exam, at completion of exam
- Assess all vital signs first
- Perform physical assessment in a head to toe sequence
- Provide privacy, drape child as each area is assessed
- Stress normal findings
- Discuss results with child/parent
- Provide educational background
- Answer all questions and concerns, inform of use of information
- Inform if any further examination needed
- Invite to participate in care plan if interested

Adolescent
- Introduce self, establish rapport
- Determine whether client wants parent in exam room
- Explain each procedure and teen-ager's role in assisting with examination
- Encourage questions, comments or concerns to be mentioned throughout exam

- Provide for privacy
- Perform assessment in a head-to-toe process
- Stress normal findings
- Perform genital exam at end of assessment; talk/explain procedure in quiet voice as each area palpated and inspected
- Answer all questions and concerns, inform of use of information
- Inform if any further examination needed
- Invite to participate in care plan if interested
- Provide educational information to adolescent and parent prn

APPENDIX F

Physical Assessment

Vital Signs

Temperature
Pulse
Respiration
Blood pressure

Measurements

Height/length
Weight
Head and chest circumference (if age appropriate)

General Condition

Appearance
Behavior
Activity
Nutrition
Hygiene

Skin

Color
Moisture
Texture
Temperature
Turgor
Hair
Nails
Lesions (color, distribution, shape, configuration, sensations)

Lymph nodes

Palpable nodes
Size
Tenderness
Shape
Mobility
Normal findings include: palpable nodes not greater than 3 mm
except in cervical and groin area where may be 1 cm

Head

Shape
Masses
Size
Symmetry
Fontanels
Sutures
Lesions
Position of eyes, ears, nose and mouth
Abnormalities

Eyes

Shape
Symmetry
Lids
Lashes
Moisture
Coordination (nystagmus or strabismus)
Exudate
PEARLA
Visual acuity

Ears

Placement
Shape
Drainage
Masses
Lesions
Foreign bodies
Tympanic membrane (light reflex - pull ear down and back in children
under the age of three)

Nose

Placement
Patency
Lesions
Drainage
Masses
Respiratory effort
Obstruction

Mouth

Color

Moisture

Lesions

Lips

Placement and size of internal structures (tongue, uvula, palates, teeth)

Number and appearance of teeth

Color of mucosa

Odor

Throat

Color

Tonsils

Exudate

Neck

Symmetry

Masses

ROM

Webbing

Pulsations

Size of thyroid

Chest

Shape

Masses

Bilateral symmetry

Pulsations

Respiratory effort and type (diaphragmatic or abdominal breathing)

Breast development and placement

Lungs

Breath sounds (intensity, quality, duration)

Sounds on inspiration and/or expiration (clear, crackles, rhonchi, wheezing, pleural rub)

Bilaterally equal chest expansion

Heart

Pulses equal in rate and intensity in all extremities

Temperature and color of extremities

Heart sounds (rate, rhythm, murmurs)

PMI
Clubbing
Palpations
Activity level
Edema

Abdomen

Size
Shape
Symmetry
Masses
Visible peristaltic activity
Bowel sounds
Appearance of umbilicus
Abdominal girth
Tenderness
Rigidity
Guarding
Rebound tenderness
Palpable liver
Spleen
Bladder
Kidney

Genitalia

Female:
Presence and position of urethra, labia, vagina
Exudate
Lesions
Masses
Pubic development/Tanner's stage
Male:
Position and shape of penis
Urethra
Scrotum
Testes
Exudate
Lesions
Masses
Pubic development/Tanner's stage

Rectum/Anus

Patency
Lesions
Muscle tone
Stools
Masses

Musculoskeletal

Gait
Posture
Stance
Coordination
Symmetry in muscle size and tone
Strength
Masses
Spinal alignment
Pilonidal dimples
Long bone alignment
Joints (ROM, tenderness, warmth, edema)
Dislocations
Hand/palm/foot appearance (palmar/plantar creases, webbing of
fingers, number of fingers/toes)

Nervous system

Alertness
Activity level
Coordination
Motor development
Cranial nerves
Reflexes
Cerebellar functions
Sensory functions

APPENDIX G

Medication Tables

The following medication charts include the commonly-prescribed medications for children. In addition to dosages specific to pediatrics, the author has placed special emphasis on nursing actions and patient teaching.

Table 1. ANALGESICS AND SEDATIVES

Name	Uses	Route and Dose	Adverse Reactions/ Side Effects	Drug or Food Interactions	Nursing Considerations
Generic: Acetaminophen **Trade:** Tylenol, Tempra	Nonnarcotic analgesic/antipyretic used for relief of mild to moderate pain and control of fever.	**PO:** **< 3 mo:** 40 mg **4 - 11 mo:** 80 mg **1 - 2 yrs:** 120 mg **2 - 3 yrs:** 160 mg **4 - 5 yrs:** 240 mg **6 - 8 yrs:** 320 mg **9 - 10 yrs:** 400 mg **11 yrs:** 480 mg **> 11 yrs:** 325 - 650 mg; not to exceed 4 g/day for short term therapy or 2.6 g/day for long term therapy **These doses may be repeated q 4 - 6 hrs PRN but should not exceed 5 doses/day or be given longer than 5 days without seeking medical advice.	**CNS:** Mental confusion, lethargy, seizures **Hepatic:** Liver damage with abnormal liver function tests within 2 - 4 days of overdose **GU:** Hematuria, renal damage and dysfunction (more common in children with renal disease). **Skin:** Rash, urticaria **Hemic:** Bleeding, ecchymosis, anemia, thrombocytopenia, leukopenia (more common with long term use) **Other:** Anaphylaxis	**Drugs:** Alcohol and other hepatotoxic drugs; decreased action with chronic barbiturate use; increased anticoagulant effect of coumarin with chronic use; increased nephrotoxicity if combined with long term aspirin use; potential for hypothermia if used with phenothiazines. **Food:** Decreased absorption if taken with a high carbohydrate meal.	• Note hepatic and renal function and monitor if long-term use anticipated. • May be crushed and given with food. • Patient/parent education includes: - Do not give with any other OTC medication. - If illness lasts > 3 days or no relief obtained, consult MD. - Limit to 5 doses/day.
Generic: Chloral Hydrate **Trade:** Aquachloral, Noctec	Hypnotic used preoperatively to reduce anxiety, postoperatively with analgesics, and for sedation prior to tests such as CT scan and MRI.	**PO, PR:** **Hypnotic:** 50 mg/kg or 1.5 g/m², not to exceed 1 g/dose **Sedative:** 8/3 mg/kg or 250 mg/m² TID; not to exceed 500 mg TID **Premedication sedation for diagnostic tests:** 20 - 25 mg/kg	**CNS:** Continued sedation, disorientation, paranoia, paradoxical excitement, headache **CV:** Dysrhythmias with overdose, bradycardia **Respiratory:** Depression with overdose **Hepatic:** Jaundice with overdose **Hemic:** Leukopenia, eosinophilia	**Drugs:** CNS depressants potentiate this medication; causes diaphoresis, flushing, and hypertension when given with IV furosemide; hypoprothrombinemia when given with oral anticoagulants, particularly warfarin **Food:** None	• Obtain baseline vital signs. • PO may be given with food to decrease gastric distress. • Check anal area prior to administering PR dose. • Put side rails up after administration and keep potentially dangerous items away from patient. • Observe for onset of sleep. • Monitor for signs of overdose. (hypotension, weakness, coma, dysrhythmias, vomiting). • Patient/parent education: - Avoid driving and performing other potentially dangerous tasks while taking this medication. - Avoid taking with other medications unless directed by physician.

Name	Uses	Route and Dose	Adverse Reactions/ Side Effects	Drug or Food Interactions	Nursing Considerations
Generic: Codeine **Trade:** Combined with other products such as Tylenol, phenergan, and guiatussin	Narcotic analgesic, opiate agonist, antitussive used to treat mild to moderate pain and suppress cough.	PO is available as codeine sulfate IM and SC are available as codeine phosphate **PO, IM, SC:** **Pain:** 3 mg/kg or 100 mg/m² in 6 divided doses; or 0.5 mg/kg or 15 mg/m² q 4 - 6h **PO:** **Antitussive:** **2 - 6 yrs:** 1 mg/kg/day in 4 doses not to more than q 4 - 6h **6 - 11 yrs:** 5 - 10 mg q 4 - 6h; not to exceed 60 mg/day **12 yrs and older:** 10 - 20 mg q 4 - 6h; not to exceed 120 mg/day	**CNS:** Sedation, restlessness, insomnia **CV:** Circulatory depression, orthostatic hypotension, palpitation, brady- or tachycardia **GI:** Nausea, vomiting, constipation **Resp:** Respiratory depression is a serious side effect **Hepatic:** Biliary spasm, increased serum amylase and lipase **GU:** Urinary retention, oliguria, impotence **Skin:** Rash, erythema, urticaria, pruritus, facial flushing	**Drug:** Potentiated by CNS depressants such as alcohol; incompatible with aminophylline, heparin, methicillin, phenobarbital, sodium bicarbonate; decreases effects of diuretics in congestive heart failure. **Food:** None	• Assess type and degree of pain prior to administration. • Use other pain control methods in addition to analgesics. • Take baseline vital signs. • Give PO forms with food to decrease gastric distress. • Rotate injection sites. • Raise side rails. • Monitor vital signs q 15 - 30 minutes following administration. • Evaluate amount of pain within 30 minutes following administration. • Patient/parent education: - Take drug only as directed and only for patient prescribed . - Drug may cause drowsiness - avoid driving and adjust other activities accordingly. - Do not administer to child < 1 yr or extended release forms to child < 6 yr. - Observe for excessive drowsiness.

Name	Uses	Route and Dose	Adverse Reactions/ Side Effects	Drug or Food Interactions	Nursing Considerations
Generic: Diazepam **Trade:** Valium	Sedative and anticonvulsant used as an anti-anxiety agent and to treat generalized seizures.	**PO:** Sedative or muscle relaxant: 0.12 - 0.8 mg/kg/day equally divided q 6 - 8 h **IM, IV:** Sedative or muscle relaxant: 0.04 - 0.2 mg/kg/dose q 2 - 4 h (max dose = 0.6 mg/kg within 8 h) Status epilepticus: 1 mo - 5 yrs: 0.2 mg/kg/dose IV q 15 - 30 min. (max. dose = 10 mg). May repeat 2 - 4 h prn.	**CNS:** Drowsiness, paradoxical excitement, dizziness, ataxia, confusion, weakness, tremor, vertigo, syncope **CV:** Hypotension, brady-cardia, cardiac arrest with rapid IV infusion **GI:** Nausea, vomiting, constipation, diarrhea, appetite and weight changes, in-creased salivation, metallic taste, decreased gag reflex **Resp:** Apnea with rapid IV infusion **GU:** Retention, incontinence **Skin:** Rash, urticaria, pruritus, photosensitivity **Musculoskeletal:** Bone pain, muscle cramps, paraesthesia **Sensory:** Blurred vision, nystagmus, diplopia	**Drugs:** Increased CNS depressant effects if given with other CNS depressants; lowered seizure threshold with tricyclic antidepressants; decreased clearance and increased levels if taken with cimetidine and disulfiram; increased hypotension with other drugs that have this effect; decreased absorption with antacids; reduced digoxin excretion; enhanced excretion with refampin; increased phenytoin levels; potentiate MAO inhibitors. **Food:** None	• Take baseline vital signs. • May give po forms with a small amount of food. • Incompatible with other drugs - do not mix if giving IV. • Interacts with plastic - give as close to vein as is possible. • Avoid extravasation. • Monitor CBC, liver function tests, nutrition and weight if on long term therapy. • Patient/parent education: - Take drug only as directed and only for patient prescribed . - Drug may cause drowsiness - avoid driving, adjust other activities accordingly. - Avoid OTC drugs, alcohol, other illicit drugs. - Report drowsiness, dizziness, excitement or other unusual effects to MD. - Wear identification if taking this medication for seizure control.
Generic: Fentanyl Citrate **Trade:** Sublimaze	Acts as a general anesthetic in higher doses and as analgesic for moderate to severe pain in lower doses.	**IV:** 1 - 4 mcg/kg/dose slow IV push repeated q 2 - 4 h prn.	**CNS:** Dizziness, sedation, weakness, restlessness, insomnia, seizures **CV:** Bradycardia, hypotension **GI:** Nausea, vomiting, abdominal cramps, constipation **Resp:** Respiratory depression, atelectasis, dyspnea **GU:** Oliguria, urinary retention **Skin:** Itching, rash, hives	**Drugs:** Potentiated by other drugs having the same effect; increased hypotensive effect with antihypertensives; benzodiazepines may increase amount of fentanyl needed; excitement and hypertension if given within 14 days of MAO inhibitors. **Food:** None	• Obtain baseline vital signs and reassess frequently with particular attention paid to respiratory rate and effort. • Patient/parent education: - Cough and deep breath frequently. - Stay in bed with side rails up.

Name	Uses	Route and Dose	Adverse Reactions/ Side Effects	Drug or Food Interactions	Nursing Considerations
Generic: Ibuprofen **Trade:** Motrin, PediaProfen	Nonsteroidal antiinflammatory, analgesic, antipyretic used for mild to moderate pain, control of fever, and to treat rheumatoid arthritis.	Safety in children under 6 mo. not established PO: **Juvenile rheumatoid arthritis:** **< 20 kg:** 400 mg/day **20 - 30 kg:** 600 mg/day **30 - 40 kg:** 800 mg/day **> 40 kg:** Adult dosage of 400 - 800 mg TID or QID but not to exceed 3.2 g/day **Fever control 6 mo - 12 yrs:** **< 39 degrees C:** 5 mg/kg **> 39 degrees C:** 10 mg/kg Maximum daily dose for fever control is 40 mg/day.	**CNS:** Dizziness, headache, confusion, depression **CV:** Fluid retention, CHF, hypertension, palpation, dysrhythmias **GI:** Nausea, vomiting, heartburn **Resp:** Bronchospasm, dyspnea **Hepatic:** Jaundice, hepatitis, altered liver enzymes **GU:** Polyuria, hematuria, renal failure **Hemic:** Inhibited platelet action, prolonged bleeding time, neutropenia, thrombocytopenia, anemia **Sensory:** Blurred or disturbed vision, tinnitus	**Drugs:** Increased renal side effects with acetaminophen and diuretics; increased risk of GI side effects with drugs having similar side effects such as corticosteroids; potentiation of anticoagulant effects when given with other drugs having same effect; hypoglycemia with insulin; decreased effect of antihypertensives; increased serum lithium levels; not recommended with any other nonsteroidal antiinflammatory drugs. **Foods:** None	• Assess for prior allergy to aspirin or other nonsteroidal antiinflammatory drugs. • Patients with asthma at higher risk for allergy. • Assess for visual disturbances and bleeding disorders. • Administration with food may decrease GI discomfort. • Monitor BUN, creatinine, SGOT, SGPT, and serum K+ levels in patients with renal or hepatic dysfunction. • Monitor bleeding time in patients with bleeding disorders. • If visual disturbances occur, eye exam as necessary. • Patient/parent education: - OTC doses are not intended for home management of pain. - Give with food to decrease GI discomfort. - Avoid alcohol and other OTC drugs. - Report rash, flu-like symptoms, visual changes, and/or yellowing of skin.

Name	Uses	Route and Dose	Adverse Reactions/Side Effects	Drug or Food Interactions	Nursing Considerations
Generic: Lorazepam **Trade:** Ativan	Used for preoperative sedation, conscious sedation, induction and maintenance of anesthesia, and relief of anxiety	**IV:** 0.05 - 0.1 mg/kg slow IV push	**CNS:** Drowsiness, sedation, dizziness, weakness, unsteadiness, disorientation, depression, sleep disturbance, restlessness, confusion, hallucinations **CV:** Hyper- or hypotension **GI:** Nausea, vomiting, abdominal discomfort, anorexia **Sensory:** Blurred vision, diplopia, depressed hearing	**Drugs:** Added depressant effects when used with other CNS depressants. **Foods:** None	• Assess vital signs prior to administration. • Assess airway patency prior to IV administration. • Dilute IV doses with an equal volume prior to administration. • Avoid giving this drug intraarterially as it may lead to gangrene and amputation. • Refrigerate parenteral preparations. • Patient/parent education: - Avoid other OTC medications unless approved by MD. - Instruct patient that amnesia may follow a preoperative dose of this drug. - Avoid alcohol. - Avoid caffeine as it counteracts this drug.
Generic: Meperidine **Trade:** Demerol, Mepergan	Narcotic analgesic used for relief of moderate to severe pain and as a preoperative medication to enhance effects of anesthesia.	**PO,IM,SC:** **Pain:** 1.1 - 1.8 mg/kg q 3 - 4 h PRN; single dose not to exceed 100 mg **IM,SC:** **Preoperative medication:** 1 - 2.2 mg/kg 30 - 90 minute before surgery; not to exceed 100 mg	**CNS:** Sedation, dizziness, depression, coma, euphoria, restlessness, insomnia **CV:** Circulatory depression, orthostatic hypotension, palpitation, bradycardia, tachycardia (more common than with other opiates) **GI:** Nausea, vomiting, constipation **Resp:** Respiratory depression **Hepatic:** Biliary spasm, increased serum amylase and lipase **GU:** Urinary retention, oliguria, impotence **Skin:** Rash, erythema, urticaria, pruritus, facial flushing	**Drugs:** Potentiated CNS effects with other CNS depressants; phenothiazines may antagonize action; may potentiate neuromuscular-blocking agents; may decrease effects of diuretics used in CHF; do not give within 14 days of MAO inhibitors; incompatible with aminophylline, heparin, methicillin, phenobarbital, sodium bicarbonate. **Food:** None	• Assess type and degree of pain. • Baseline vital signs. • Evaluate pain relief/control within 30 minutes of administration. • Patient/parent education: - Take only as directed and only for patient prescribed. - Produces altered mental alertness, therefore, avoid driving and adjust other activities as necessary.

Name	Uses	Route and Dose	Adverse Reactions/ Side Effects	Drug or Food Interactions	Nursing Considerations
Generic: Midazolam Hydrochloride **Trade:** Versed	Benzodiazepine used to reduce anxiety, as a muscle relaxant, and as an amnesiac. Also used for induction of general anesthesia and to reduce anxiety prior to diagnostic tests such as CT scan.	**IV,IM:** 0.07 - 0.2 mg/kg; repeat as required, usually q 2 - 4h. Continuous infusion: Bolus 0.2 mg/kg to be followed by a 0.3 - 0.5 mcg/kg/minute infusion.	**CNS:** Excessive sedation, drowsiness, paradoxical excitement, hyperactivity, anxiety, restlessness, confusion **CV:** Hypotension, bradycardia, tachycardia **GI:** Nausea, vomiting, increased salivation, dry mouth, constipation **Resp:** Decreased respiratory rate, apnea **Skin:** Pain at injection site, urticaria, rash, pruritus **Sensory:** Blurred vision, diplopia, nystagmus, blocked ears	**Drugs:** Potentiated with other CNS depressants; potentiated by cimetidine or ranitidine. **Food:** None	• Baseline vital signs. • Provide for patient safety following administration (raise side rails, etc.). • Place patient on cardiac/respiratory monitor if administering IV and have emergency equipment available. • Monitor blood pressure for hypotension. • Monitor for respiratory depression. • Patient/parent education: - Avoid other CNS depressants when taking this medication.
Generic: Morphine Sulfate **Trade:** Morphine	Narcotic analgesic used for treatment of severe pain and preoperatively.	**PO:** 0.3 mg/kg q 4h **IV,IM,SC:** 0.1 - 0.2 mg/kg/dose repeated q 2 - 4h PRN, not to exceed 15 mg/dose **Continuous Infusion (PCA Pump):** 0.04 - 0.07 mg/kg/hour **Epidural Infusion:** Established by practitioner based on the patient's pain level and weight (three "p's")	**CNS:** Sedation, coma, dizziness, depression, euphoria, restlessness, insomnia **CV:** Circulatory depression, orthostatic hypotension, bradycardia, tachycardia **GI:** Nausea, vomiting, constipation **Resp:** Respiratory depression **Hepatic:** Biliary spasm, increased serum amylase and lipase **GU:** Urinary retention, oliguria, impotence **Skin:** Rash, erythema, urticaria, pruritus, facial flushing	**Drugs:** Potentiated by other CNS depressants; antagonized by phenothiazines; may decreased effects of diuretics in CHF. **Food:** None	• Obtain baseline vital signs, particularly respiratory rate. • Assess type and amount of pain. • Monitor vital signs q 15 - 30 minutes following administration. • Assess effectiveness 30 minutes following administration. • Have naloxone available to treat side effects (including itching as it is a side effect of the morphine and not histamine related). • Provide for patient safety (side rails up, etc.). • Patient/parent education: - This medication should be used only as directed and only for patient prescribed. - Report any side effects such as itching or nausea and administer naloxone as ordered.

Table 2. ANTIBIOTICS

Name	Uses	Route and Dose	Adverse Reactions/ Side Effects	Drug or Food Interactions	Nursing Considerations
Generic: Amikacin **Trade:** Amikin	Aminoglycoside active against gram + and gram - bacteria used for treatment of infections of bone, burns, urinary tract, and CNS and for septicemia and otitis media.	**IV,IM:** **Neonates < 7 days:** **< 28 weeks:** 7.5 mg/kg/ dose q 24h **28 - 34 weeks:** 7.5 mg/kg/ dose q 18h **Term:** 7.5 mg/kg/dose q 12h **Neonates > 7 days:** **< 28 weeks:** 7.5 mg/kg/ dose q 18h **28 - 34 weeks:** 7.5 mg/kg/ dose q 12h **Term:** 7.5 mg/kg/dose q 8h **Children:** 15 mg/kg/day q 8h with a maximum dose of 1.5 gm/day Infusion rate for infants is over 1 - 2h and children is over 30 - 60 minutes.	**CNS:** Neurotoxicity, neuromuscular blockade, numbness, tingling, muscle twitching, seizures, lethargy **GI:** Nausea, vomiting, loss of appetite **GU:** Nephrotoxicity, blood in urine, oliguria, proteinuria **Skin:** Rash, drug fever **Hemic:** Eosinophilia, anemia **Sensory:** Ototoxicity	**Drug:** Increased chance of ototoxicity if used with other aminoglycosides and capreomycin. Ototoxicity and nephrotoxicity chances increased if used with Amphotericin B, salicylates, bacitracin (parenteral), bumetanide (parenteral), carmustine, cephalothin, cisplatin, cyclosporine, etha-crynic acid, furosemide, paromomycin, streptozocin, vancomycin. Increases respiratory depressant effects of opoids and anal-gesics. Inactivated by peni-cillin, carbicillin, and ticarcillin. **Food:** None	* Culture and sensitivity should be ob-tained prior to starting treatment. * Do not give IV push. * Do not use solution if it is dark yel-low or has particulate matter. * Dilute to maximum amount. * Monitor hearing. * Assess renal function by monitoring I&O, daily weights, urine specific gravity, UA, creatinine levels, and BUN.

Name	Uses	Route and Dose	Adverse Reactions/ Side Effects	Drug or Food Interactions	Nursing Considerations
Generic: - Amoxicillin - Amoxicillin with Clavulanate potassium **Trade:** Amoxil (without clavulanate potassium) Augmentin (with clavulanate potassium)	Antibiotic used to treat infections of ear, respiratory tract, urinary tract, and skin and soft tissue.	**PO:** **< 20 kg:** 20 - 40 mg/kg/day divided q 8h **> 20 kg:** 250 - 500 mg divided q 8h Adjust dose in patients with renal impairment	**GI:** Diarrhea (more common with clavulanate potassium), nausea, vomiting (common with clavulanate potassium), epigastric pain, stomatitis, glossitis **Hepatic:** Moderate rise in SGOT and SGPT **GU:** Superinfections (primarily yeast), interstitial nephritis **Skin:** Erythematous, maculopapular, mildly pruritic rash **Hemic:** Anemia, thrombocytopenia, thrombocytopenic purpura, agranulocytosis, leukopenia, eosinophilia	**Drugs:** Erythromycin, tetracycline, chloromycetin, and acids. Probenecid decreases renal excretion and prolongs serum levels. **Food:** None	* Assess for previous allergy to amoxicillin, penicillin, cephalosporins. * Assess for asthma and family history of allergies. * Monitor for hypersensitivity reaction (first 20 minutes). * Monitor for signs of superinfection. * Patient/parent education: - Finish all medication. - Note any side effects and report to physician. - Reconstituted suspension should be discarded after 14 days.

Name	Uses	Route and Dose	Adverse Reactions/ Side Effects	Drug or Food Interactions	Nusrsing Considerations
Generic: Ampicillin **Trade:** Omnipen Polycillin	Broad spectrum antibiotic used to treat infections of the ear, meninges, upper respiratory tract, GU tract, skin and soft tissue.	**PO:** 50 - 100 mg/kg/day equally divided q 6h **IV,IM:** **Neonates:** **< 7 days:** 50 - 100 mg/kg/day divided q 12h **> 7 days:** 100 - 200 mg/kg/day divided q 8 h **Mild - moderate infections:** 50 - 100 mg/kg/day divided q 6 h **Severe infections:** 200 - 400 mg/kg/day divided q 4 - 6h	**CNS:** Seizures (usually seen in excess of 400 mg/kg/day) **Gi:** Diarrhea, nausea, vomiting, epigastric pain, pseudomembranous colitis, stomatitis, glossitis, black tongue **Hepatic:** Moderate rise in SGOT **GU:** Superinfections primarily yeast **Skin:** Erythematous, maculopapular, mildly pruritus rash **Hemic:** Eosinophilia, anemia, thrombocytopenia, thrombocy-topenic purpura, leukopenia, agranulocytosis	**Drugs:** Erythromycin, tetracycline, chloramphenicol decrease effects; allopurinol may enhance development of rash; may interfere with effectiveness of oral contraceptives **Food:** Absorption hampered by food	* Assess for previous allergy to drug, penicillins, cephalosporins, other drugs, asthma, or family history of allergies. * Obtain culture and sensitivity prior to beginning treatment. * Give 1 hr prior or 2 hrs following meals. * Reconstitute with sterile or bacteriostatic water. * Do not use bacteriostatic preparations containing benzyl alcohol with neonates. * Do not exceed IV rate of 100 mg/minute. * Stability decreases with dextrose. * Observe for signs of hypersensitivity (first 20 min after first dose) or superinfection. * Patient/parent education: - Finish all medication. - Monitor for side effects and report rash or diarrhea to physician. - May interfere with effectiveness of oral contraceptives.
Generic: Cefaclor **Trade:** Ceclor	Second generation cephalosporin used to treat otitis media, respiratory, urinary tract and skin infections.	**PO:** > 1 mo: 20 - 40 mg/kg/day divided q 8 - 12h	**CNS:** Headache, dizziness **GI:** Diarrhea, nausea, vomiting, anorexia, cramps, heartburn **GU:** Increased BUN and serum creatinine, vaginitis **Hemic:** Increased SGOT, SGPT, alkaline phosphatase	**Drugs:** None noted **Food:** Food decreases absorption time.	* Assess for previous allergy to drug, penicillins, cephalosporins, other drugs, asthma, or family history of allergies. * Obtain culture and sensitivity prior to beginning treatment. * Medication is expensive - use only with susceptible organisms. * Monitor for superinfection. * Patient/parent education: - Finish all medication. - Observe for side effects. - Store suspension in refrigerator and discard after 14 days.

Name	Uses	Route and Dose	Adverse Reactions/ Side Effects	Drug or Food Interactions	Nursing Considerations
Generic: Cefazolin **Trade:** Kefzol Ancef	First generation cephalosporin used to treat respiratory, biliary and GU tract, skin, bone and joint infections, septicemia, and endocarditis.	IM,IV: **< 7 days:** 40 mg/kg/day divided q 12h **1 - 4 wks:** 60 mg/kg/day divided q 8h **> 1 mo:** 25 - 100 mg/kg/day divided q 8h **Maximum dose:** 6 g/day Adjust dose in renal impairment	**GI:** <u>Pseudomembranous colitis</u>, anorexia, diarrhea, thrush, abdominal cramps, nausea, vomiting **GU:** Transient rise in BUN, SGOT, SGPT and alkaline phosphatase, pruritus, genital moniliasis, vaginitis **Hemic:** Transient neutropenia, leukopenia, <u>thrombocytopenia</u>	**Drugs:** Combination with probenecid inhibits renal excretion, thus prolonging serum levels; aminoglycosides, chloramphenicol, and penicillins may cause synergistic effects. **Food:** None	• Assess for previous allergy to cefa-zolin, cephalosporins, and penicillins. • Obtain culture and sensitivity prior to starting medication. • Monitor for hypersensitivity, symptoms of superinfection, and diarrhea.
Generic: Cefotaxime **Trade:** Claforan	Third generation cephalosporin used to treat infections of lower respiratory tract, skin, GU tract, bone, joint, and septicemias, gynecologic, CNS infections, and gonococcal ophthalmic infections.	IV,IM: **Neonates:** **< 7 days:** 50 - 100 mg/kg/day q 12h **1 - 4 wks:** 50 - 150 mg/kg/day q 8h **1 - 12 yrs:** **< 50 kg:** 50 - 180 mg/kg/day divided q 4 - 6h **> 50 kg:** 1 - 2 g q 6 - 8h (Maximum dose 10 - 12 g/day) Adjust dose for renal impairment	**CNS:** Headache **GI:** <u>Pseudomembranous colitis</u>, diarrhea, nausea, vomiting **Hepatic:** Transient rise of SGOT, SGPT, serum LDH, serum alkaline phosphatase **GU:** Transient rise BUN, moniliasis, vaginitis **Skin:** Maculopapular or erythematous rash, pruritus, fever **Hemic:** <u>Granulocytopenia</u>, transient eosinophilia, leukopenia, neutropenia, <u>thrombocytopenia</u>	**Drugs:** Probenecid inhibits renal excretion, thus prolonging serum levels; synergistic effects with certain organisms when combined with aminoglycosides, chloramphenicol, and penicillins; nephrotoxicity increased with concomitant administration of aminoglycosides, potassium-depleting diuretics, and other cephalosporins. **Food:** None	• Assess for previous allergy to cefotaxime, penicillins, or cephalosporins. • Obtain culture and sensitivity prior to starting medication. • IM injection painful. • Do not premix with other aminoglycosides, aminophylline, sodium bicarbonate, or alkaline solutions. • Monitor for hypersensitivity and side effects.

Name	Uses	Route and Dose	Adverse Reactions Side Effects	Drug or Food Interactions	Nursing Considerations
Generic: Clindamycin **Trade:** Cleocin	Antibiotic used against gram + bacterial infections and to treat acne vulgaris.	**PO:** < 10 kg: 37.5 mg q 8h > 10 kg: 8 - 25 mg/kg/day q 6 - 8h **IM,IV:** **Preterm and small neonates:** 15 mg/kg/day **< 1 mo:** 15 - 20 mg/kg/day q 6 - 8 h **> 1 mo:** 15 - 40 mg/kg/day q 6 - 8h **Topical:** Apply thin film BID	**GI:** <u>Pseudomembranous colitis</u>, diarrhea, nausea, vomiting, abdominal pain, flatulence, esophagitis **Hepatic:** Transient rise of SGOT, serum bilirubin, alkaline phosphatase **GU:** Azotemia, oliguria, proteinuria **Skin:** Topical: dryness, erythema, burning, peeling, pruritus **Hemic:** Transient leukopenia, neutropenia, thrombocytopenia, eosinophilia, agranulocytosis **Musculoskeletal:** Polyarthritis **Other:** Hypersensitivity (maculopapular rash, urticaria, pruritus erythema multiforme); local: IM - pain, induration, sterile abscess; IV - pain, edema, erythema, thrombophlebitis, <u>hypotension and cardiac arrest if infused too rapidly</u>	**Drugs:** May potentiate neuromuscular blocking agents such as pancuronium and atracurium, possible antagonism with aminoglycosides **Foods:** None	• Assess for previous allergy to this drug or lincomycin. • Obtain culture and sensitivity prior to starting medication. • Obtain baseline hematological, renal, and hepatic studies prior to beginning long term therapy. • Observe and report appearance of skin with topical use. • Do not refrigerate po solutions. • May give with food. • If given po, encourage fluids to avoid esophagitis. • <u>IM injection is painful - do not give 600 mg per injection site.</u> • Do not give IV push. • Dilute IV doses to a minimum of 6 mg/ml and give no faster than 30 mg/minute. • Avoid eye area with topical applications. • Monitor IM injection sites for induration and abscess. • Monitor IV sites for extravasation and thrombophlebitis. • Monitor for superinfection, primarily yeast. • Patient/parent education: - Teach proper application of topical solution. - Emphasize strict adherence to oral dosing schedule. - Stress need for continued close medical supervision during therapy. - Report any adverse reactions (especially diarrhea) to MD.

Name	Uses	Route and Dose	Adverse Reactions/ Side Effects	Drug or Food Interactions	Nursing Considerations
Generic: Co-Trimoxazole **Trade:** Bactrim	Wide-spectrum antibiotic. Not effective against *Pseudomonas*, enterococci, mycobacteria, or *Clostridia*.	**PO,IV: Minor infections:** **< 40 kg:** 8 - 10 mg/kg/day divided q 12h **> 40 kg:** 320 mg/day divided q 12h **Severe infections:** 20 mg/kg/day divided q 6 - 8h	**CNS:** Headache, lethargy, ataxia, nervousness **GI:** Nausea, vomiting, pain, stomatitis, <u>pseudomembranous</u> <u>enterocolitis</u>, pancreatitis **Hepatic:** <u>Hepatitis</u> **GU:** Increased BUN and creatinine, crystalluria **Skin:** Erythematous, maculopapular, morbilliform rashes, urticaria **Hemic:** <u>Agranulocytosis,</u> <u>aplastic anemia, leuko-</u> <u>penia, neutropenia, throm-</u> <u>bocytopenia, hemolytic</u> <u>anemia</u> **Other:** <u>Epidermal necro-</u> <u>lysis, Steven-Johnson</u> <u>syndrome, exfoliative</u> <u>dermatitis, allergic</u> <u>myocarditis, anaphylaxis</u>	**Drugs:** Use with warfarin may prolong prothrombin time; may displace metho- trexate binding sites when used in combination; interferes with bactericidal effects of penicillins; may interfere with hepatic metabolism of phenytoin. **Foods:** May slightly delay absorption - give on empty stomach.	* Assess for previous allergy to sul- fonamides. * Obtain culture and sensitivity prior to starting medication. * Give on empty stomach, if possible. * Do not give IV push or rapid infusion * Keep well hydrated. * Observe for adverse reactions/side effects. * Patient/parent education: - Finish all medication. - Observe for side effects. - Maintain hydration. - Protect from sun as this may cause a hypersensitivity reaction.

Name	Uses	Route and Dose	Adverse Reactions/ Side Effects	Drug or Food Interactions	Nursing Considerations
Generic: Dicloxacillin sodium

Trade: Pathocil | Antibiotic that is the drug of choice for oral use in treating penicillinase-producing *Staphylococcus aureus* and *S. epidermidis* infections. | **PO:**
> 1 mo:
< 40 kg: 12.5 - 25 mg/kg/day equally divided q 6h
> 40 kg: 125 - 250 mg q 6h | **GI:** Nausea, vomiting, epigastric pain, loose stools, diarrhea, flatulence, hemorrhagic colitis
Hepatic: Transient rise in SGOT, SGPT
Skin: Rashes, pruritus indicating hypersensitivity
Hemic: Eosinophilia, anemia, neutropenia, thrombocytopenia, leukopenia
Other: Hypersensitivity indicated by drug fever | **Drugs:** Erythromycin, tetracycline, chloromycetin decrease antibacterial effects.

Food: Food interferes with absorption of this medication. | • Assess for previous allergy to drug, penicillins, cephalosporins, other drugs, asthma, other allergies.
• Obtain culture and sensitivity prior to starting medication.
• Give on empty stomach (1 hour prior or 2 hours following meals) as food interferes with absorption.
• Refrigerate solution and shake well.
• Monitor for hypersensitivity, rash, and other side effects.
• Maintain fluid intake.
• Patient/parent education:
- Finish all medication.
- Observe for side effects such as diarrhea.
- Do not take OTC drugs without consulting MD.
- Store solution in refrigerator out of reach of children and discard after 14 days. |

Name	Uses	Route and Dose	Adverse Reactions/ Side Effects	Drug or Food Interactions	Nursing Considerations
Generic: Erythromycin **Trade:** E-Mycin **Generic:** Erythromycin ethylsuccinate **Trade:** E.E.S. Pediamycin **Generic:** Erythromycin estolate **Trade:** Ilosone	Antibiotic active against gram + and - bacteria used to treat infections of respiratory tract, skin, soft tissue, otitis media, Lyme disease, neonatal conjunctivitis and ocular infections, acne and superficial wounds.	**PO:** 30 - 50 mg/kg/day equally divided q 6 - 8h Prophylaxis rheumatic fever: 500 mg BID **IV:** 10 - 20 mg/kg/day equally divided q 6h **Ophthalmic:** Prophylaxis neonatal gonococcal ophthalmia: Instill 0.5 - 2 cm strip into conjunctival sac within 1 hour post delivery **Combination form:** Pediazole: > 2 months: 50 mg erythromycin and 150 mg sulfisoxazole/kg/day equally divided q 6h	**GI:** Abdominal pain and cramping, nausea, vomiting, diarrhea, stomatitis, anorexia **Skin:** Dryness, erythema, burning, peeling **Sensory:** Tinnitus, vertigo, ototoxicity, reversible bilateral hearing loss **Other:** Anaphylaxis, urticaria, skin eruptions, rash **Local: IV:** Venous irritation, thrombophlebitis; IM causes severe pain	**Drugs:** Antagonistic action if given with clindamycin; potential toxicity if given with carbamazepine, cyclosporine, theophylline, and digoxin; increased effects if given with oral anticoagulants. **Foods:** Absorption delayed if administered with food depending upon formulation prescribed.	• Assess for previous allergy. • Obtain culture and sensitivity prior to starting medication. • Give on empty stomach. • Do not crush film or enteric-coated tablets. • May take apart time release capsules but instruct patient not to chew particles. • Do not give IV push or rapid infusion. • Give IV solution slowly as solution is irritating. • Observe for adverse reactions/side effects. • Patient/parent education: - Finish all medication. - Observe for side effects. - Teach proper administration technique.

Name	Uses	Route and Dose	Adverse Reactions/ Side Effects	Drug or Food Interactions	Nursing Considerations

Generic: Gentamycin
 	
Trade: Garamycin
	Aminoglycoside active against wide range of gram + and - bacteria. Used to treat infections of bone, skin, urinary and GI tract, neonatal and bacterial septicemias, meningitis, external eye and adnexa, primary and secondary skin infections.	**IM,IV:**
		Neonates ≤ 7 days:
		< 28 weeks: 2.5 mg/kg q 24 hrs
		28 - 34 weeks: 2.5 mg/kg q 18 hrs
		Term: 2.5 mg/kg q 12 hrs
		
		Neonates > 7 days:
		< 28 weeks: 2.5 mg/kg q 18 hrs
		28 - 34 weeks: 2.5 mg/kg q 12 hrs
		
		Infants, 7 days - 1 year: 2.5 mg/kg q 8 hrs
		> 1 year: 2 - 2.5 mg/kg q 8 hrs
		Children: 6 - 7.5 mg/kg/ day equally divided q 8 hrs
		
		Intrathecal:
		< 3 months: dosage not established
		> 3 months: 1 - 2 mg QD
		
		Ophthalmic:
		Drops: 1 drop 0.3% solution into conjunctival sac q 4 - 8 hrs
		Ointment: 1 cm strip of 0.3% ointment into conjunctival sac q 6 - 12 hrs
		
		Topical:
		0.1% sparingly applied 3 - 4 times per day
			CNS: <u>Neurotoxicity</u>, <u>neuro-muscular blockade</u>, numbness, tingling, muscle twitching and weakness, respiratory depression, lethargy, headache
			GI: Nausea, vomiting, loss of appetite
			GU: <u>Nephrotoxicity</u>, increased BUN and creatinine, <u>oliguria, renal failure</u>
			Skin: Itching, redness, edema
			Hemic: Agranulocytosis, anemia, leukopenia, eosino-philia, thrombocytopenia
			Sensory: <u>Ototoxicity</u>, hearing loss due to damage to eighth cranial nerve, tinnitus
				Drugs: Increased chance of ototoxicity and nephro-toxicity if used concurrently with amphotericin B, salicylates, parenteral bacitracin, antineoplastics, vancomycin; masked symptoms of ototoxicity if used with dimenhydrinate; increased chance of ototoxi-city if used with other aminoglycosides; increased respiratory depressant effects of opioids and analgesics; inactivated by parenteral carbenicillin and ticarcillin.
				
				Food: None
					• Assess for previous allergy.
					• Obtain culture and sensitivity prior to starting medication.
					• Obtain baseline weights, BUN and creatinine, and hearing tests.
					• Observe for respiratory depression with IV infusion.
					• Do not give IV push or rapid infusion.
					• Monitor blood levels of medication.
					• Observe for adverse reactions/side effects.
					• Discontinue therapy if no improve-ment in 3 - 5 days.
					• Monitor hearing function.
					• Patient/parent education:
					  - Finish all medication.
					  - Observe for side effects, including hearing loss.
					  - Teach proper administration tech-nique.
					  - If no improvement in 3 - 5 days, notify MD.

Name	Uses	Route and Dose	Adverse Reactions/ Side Effects	Drug or Food Interactions	Nursing Considerations
Generic: Kanamycin **Trade:** Kantrex	Aminoglycoside used to treat infections of bone, skin, urinary and GI tract and as preoperative agent for bowel surgery.	**PO,IM,IV:** **Birth - 7 days, ≤ 2000 gm:** 7.5 mg/kg q 12h **Birth - 7 days, > 2000 gm:** 7.5 mg/kg q 8 - 12h **1 - 4 weeks, ≤ 2000 gm:** 10 mg/kg q 12h **1 - 4 weeks, > 2000 gm:** 10 mg/kg q 8h **> 4 weeks:** 15 - 30 mg/kg/day equally divided q 8 - 12h	**CNS:** <u>Neurotoxicity</u>, <u>neuro-muscular blockade</u>, numbness, tingling, muscle twitching and weakness, respiratory depression, lethargy, headache **GI:** **Nausea**, vomiting, loss of appetite , <u>malabsorption syndrome</u> (long-term therapy) **GU:** <u>Nephrotoxicity</u>, increased BUN and creatinine, <u>oliguria</u>, <u>renal failure</u> **Skin:** Itching, redness, edema **Hemic:** Agranulocytosis, anemia, leukopenia, eosinophilia, thrombocytopenia **Sensory:** <u>Ototoxicity</u>, hearing loss due to damage to eighth cranial nerve, tinnitus	**Drugs:** Increased chance of ototoxicity and nephrotoxicity if used concurrently with amphotericin B, salicylates, parenteral bacitracin, antineoplastics, vancomycin; masked symptoms of ototoxicity if used with dimenhydrinate; increased chance of ototoxicity if used with other aminoglycosides; increased respiratory depressant effects of opioids and analgesics, inactivated by parenteral penicillin, carbenicillin and ticarcillin. **Food:** None	• Assess for previous allergy. • Obtain culture and sensitivity prior to starting medication. • Obtain baseline weights, BUN and creatinine, and hearing tests. • Solution may darken with age without affecting potency. • May mix with food. • If used prior to bowel surgery, dose same as for adults. • Do not give IV push or rapid infusion. • Monitor blood levels of medication. • Observe for adverse reactions/side effects. • Discontinue therapy if no improvement in 3 - 5 days. • Monitor hearing function. • Patient/parent education: - Finish all medication. - Observe for side effects, including hearing loss. - Teach proper administration technique. - If no improvement in 3 - 5 days, notify MD.

Name	Uses	Route and Dose	Adverse Reactions/ Side Effects	Drug or Food Interactions	Nursing Considerations
Generic: Methicillin **Trade:** Staphcillin	Antibiotic used to treat penicillinase-producing *Staphylococcus aureus* and *S. epidermidis* infections.	**IM,IV:** **Neonates:** **≤ 7 days:** 50 - 100 mg/kg/day equally divided q 12h **> 7 days:** 100 - 200 mg/kg/day equally divided q 6 - 8h **Children:** 100 - 400 mg/kg/day equally divided q 4 - 6 h	**GI:** Hairy tongue, oral lesions, glossitis, stomatitis **GU:** Acute interstitial nephritis with symptoms onset 5 days - 5 weeks after therapy started - usually reversible but may cause renal failure and/or death **Hepatic:** Transient rise in SGOT, SGPT, alkaline phosphatase **Skin:** Rashes, pruritus **Hemic:** Agranulocytosis, anemia, leukopenia, eosinophilia, thrombocytopenia, neutropenia **Other:** Drug fever **Local:** IM painful, sterile abscesses; IV: phlebitis, thrombophlebitis	**Drugs:** Erythromycin, tetracycline, chloramphenicol decrease antibacterial effects. **Food:** None	* Assess for previous allergy to this drug, penicillins, cephalosporins, other drugs, asthma and family history of allergies. * Obtain culture and sensitivity prior to starting medication. * Obtain baseline renal, hepatic, and hematologic tests. * Reconstituted solution may darken to deep orange following several days at room temperature - discard. * Injection is painful - give slowly and deep into large muscle. * May give slow IV push. * Change IV sites q 48 hours. * Monitor IM injection sites for sterile abscess. * Maintain hydration to prevent onset of hemorrhagic cystitis. * Observe for adverse reactions/side effects. * Patient/parent education: - Finish all medication. - Observe for side effects. - Each proper administration technique.

Name	Uses	Route and Dose	Adverse Reactions/ Side Effects	Drug or Food Interactions	Nursing Considerations
Generic: Nafcillin **Trade:** Nafcil Unipen	Antibiotic used for penicillinase-producing *Staphylococcus aureus* and *S. epidermidis* infections.	**PO:** Older infants and children: 50 - 100 mg/kg/day equally divided q 6h **IM,IV:** **Neonates ≤ 7 days:** 40 mg/kg/day equally divided q 12h **Neonates > 7 days:** 60 mg/kg/day equally divided q 6 - 8h **Older infants and children:** 100 - 200 mg/kg/day equally divided q 12h if IM or equally divided q 4h if IV	**GI:** Nausea, vomiting, diarrhea **GU:** Hematuria, dysuria, oliguria, proteinuria **Hepatic:** Transient rise in SGOT, SGPT, alkaline phosphatase **Skin:** Rashes, pruritus **Hemic:** Agranulocytosis, anemia, leukopenia, eosinophilia, thrombocytopenia, neutropenia **Other:** Serum sickness, anaphylaxis **Local:** IM painful, sterile abscesses, IV: phlebitis, thrombophlebitis, extravasation causes severe chemical irritation that can result in full thickness skin loss and gangrene	**Drugs:** Erythromycin, tetracycline, chloramphenicol decrease antibacterial effects; potentiates anticoagulants; serum concentrations increased and half-life prolonged by probenecid. **Food:** Interferes with absorption; give on empty stomach.	• Assess for previous allergy to this drug, penicillins, cephalosporins, other drugs, asthma and family history of allergies. • Obtain culture and sensitivity prior to starting medication. • Obtain baseline renal, hepatic, and hematologic tests. • Administer on empty stomach. • Injection is painful. • Monitor carefully if given IV - extravasation causes severe damage to skin and surrounding tissues . • May give slow IV push . • Change IV sites q 24 - 48 hours. • Monitor IM injection sites for sterile abscess. • Observe for adverse reactions/side effects. • Patient/parent education: - Finish all medication. - Observe for side effects. - Teach proper administration technique.

Name	Uses	Route and Dose	Adverse Reactions/ Side Effects	Drug or Food Interactions	Nursing Considerations
Generic: Nitrofurantoin **Trade:** Macrodantin Furadantin Furan	Antiinfective used primarily in UTI or prophylaxis against UTI.	**PO:** **> 1 mo:** 5 - 7 mg/kg/day equally divided q 6 hrs **Prophylaxis:** 1 - 2 mg/kg/day HS or BID	**CNS:** Peripheral neuro-pathy, headache, vertigo **GI:** Anorexia, nausea, vomiting, abdominal pain and diarrhea **Resp:** Hypersensitivity: 3 types: a). acute: severe dyspnea, chills, fever, cough, chest pain - may occur 8 hrs to 3 weeks after initiation of therapy but reversible if drug stopped; b). subacute: tachy-pnea, dyspnea, fever, cough - occurs 1 month after initiation of therapy but recovery slower; c). chronic: dyspnea on exertion, altered pulmo-nary function, malaise, cough - occurs after continuous therapy for 6 months and may cause permanent pulmonary damage **Hepatic:** Cholestatic jaundice, hepatic necrosis **GU:** Dark yellow or brown urine, crystalluria **Skin:** Erythema multiforme, exfoliative dermatitis, Stevens-Johnson syndrome, photo-sensitivity, transient alopecia **Hemic:** Agranulocytosis, leukopenia, eosinophilia, hemolytic anemia **Other:** Hypersensitivity, asthma (if previous history), anaphylaxis	**Drugs:** Renal excretion impaired and toxicity increased by probenecid and sulfinpyrazone; magnesium trisilicate antacids decrease absorption; antagonizes quinolone-derivative antiinfectives. **Food:** None	• Assess for previous allergy. • Obtain culture and sensitivity prior to starting medication. • Assess renal function. • May be mixed or given with food. • Contact with teeth may cause yellow staining. • Maintain hydration. • Observe for adverse reactions/side effects - these are not dose related. • Patient/parent education: - Finish all medication. - Observe for side effects. - Teach proper administration tech-nique. - Inform of discoloration of urine. - Stop medication and inform MD if tingling, numbness, or dyspnea occurs.

Name	Uses	Route and Dose	Adverse Reactions/ Side Effects	Drug or Food Interactions	Nursing Considerations
Generic: Rifampin **Trade:** Rifamate	Antibiotic used to treat *Mycobacterium tuberculosis, Neisseria meningitidis,* and for prophylaxis against *Haemophilus influenzae* type B.	**PO:** **Antituberculosis:** **5 yrs:** 10 - 20 mg/kg/day **Meningitis carriers or meningitis prophylaxis:** **0-1 mo:** 10 mg/kg/day QD x 4 days **>1 mo:** 20 mg/kg/day QD x 4 days ***Haemophilus Influenzae* type B prophylaxis:** **0-1 mo:** 10 mg/kg/day QD x 4 days **>1 mo:** 20 mg/kg/day QD x 4 days **Maximum dose:** 600 mg/kg/day	**CNS:** Headache, fatigue, drowsiness, ataxia, dizziness, confusion, generalized numbness **GI:** Heartburn, epigastric distress, nausea, vomiting, anorexia, diarrhea, flatulence, sore mouth and tongue **Hepatic:** Transient rise in SGPT, SGOT, alkaline phosphatase, bilirubin, <u>jaundice</u> **GU:** Hematuria, hemoglobinuria, increased BUN and serum uric acid, <u>renal insufficiency</u> **Hemic:** Thrombocytopenia, leukopenia, purpura, hemolytic anemia **Musculoskeletal:** Muscle weakness, joint and extremity pain **Other:** Reddish orange color to urine, feces, saliva, sweat and tears; hypersensitivity reaction has flu-like symptoms	**Drug:** Increased chance of hepatotoxicity with alcohol intake; causes liver enzymes to inactivate barbiturates, corticosteroids, digitalis derivatives, quinidine, dapsone, cyclosporine, chloramphenicol, oral anticoagulants, estrogens, and oral contraceptives; decreased absorption with concurrent administration of clofazimine. **Food:** Absorption may be decreased with food intake but may give with food if gastric distress.	• Obtain culture and sensitivity prior to starting medication. • Assess baseline renal and hematopoietic status. • May be mixed or given with food if gastric distress noted. • Maintain hydration. • Assess for jaundice and other side effects. • Patient/parent education: - Finish all medication as prescribed. - Observe for side effects. - Teach proper administration technique. - Inform of discoloration of body fluids. - May permanently discolor contact lens. - Maintain close medical follow-up.

Name	Uses	Route and Dose	Adverse Reactions/ Side Effects	Drug or Food Interactions	Nursing Considerations
Generic: Sulfisoxazole **Trade:** Gantrisin Combined with erythromycin ethylsuccinate to make Pediazole	Antibiotic active against both gram + and - bacteria.	**PO:** **> 2 mo:** **Loading dose:** 75 mg/kg **Maintenance:** 150 mg/kg/day equally divided q 4 - 6h (max. dose = 6 g/day) **IV:** **Loading dose:** 50 mg/kg **Maintenance:** 100 mg/kg/day q 6h **Ophthalmic:** **Drops:** 1 - 2 drops 4% solution into conjunctival sac q 8h **Ointment:** 1 cm strip into conjunctival sac q 8h	**CNS:** Headache, lethargy, nervousness, ataxia, mental depression, seizures, hallucinations **GI:** Nausea, vomiting, diarrhea, GI pain, stomatitis, pseudomembranous entero-colitis, pancreatitis **Hepatic:** Jaundice **GU:** Crystalluria, increased BUN and serum creatinine, oliguria, hematuria, proteinuria **Hemic:** Granulocytopenia, agranulocytosis, thrombocytopenia, leukopenia, hemolytic anemia, aplastic anemia, neutropenia **Sensory:** Ophthalmic itching, redness, burning, blurred vision **Other:** Epidermal necrolysis, Stevens-Johnson syndrome, exfoliative dermatitis, allergic myocarditis, serum sickness, anaphylaxis	**Drugs:** Prolonged PTT if used with coumarin; displaces protein binding sites of methotrexate, phenytoin, and salicylates; antagonized by local anesthetics. **Food:** Decreased absorption if given with food but may do so if nausea occurs.	• Assess for previous allergy to drug combination or sulfonamides. • Obtain culture and sensitivity prior to starting medication. • Assess baseline CBC, UA, renal function tests, especially if treatment > 2 weeks. • May be mixed or given with food if gastric distress noted. • Maintain hydration to prevent crystalluria. • Assess for sore throat, fever, skin rash, and sore mouth and signs of blood dyscrasias. • Patient/parent education: - Finish all medication as prescribed. - Observe for side effects. - Teach proper administration technique. - Maintain hydration levels. - Protect child from sun. - Store suspension at room temperature. - Consult MD prior to taking OTC medications.

Name	Uses	Route and Dose	Adverse Reactions/ Side Effects	Drug or Food Interactions	Nursing Considerations

Generic: Tetracycline
 	
 Trade: Panmycin Tetraclor
	Antiinfective active against a variety of gram + and - organisms although a high percentage (10 - 40%) of gram - organisms are resistant to the drug.	**PO:**
		Older infants and children: 25 - 50 mg/kg/day equally divided q 6 hrs
		> 40 kg: 1 - 2 gm/day equally divided q 6 hrs
		Chlamydia genital infections: 500 mg q 6 hrs
		
		IM:
		Older infants and children: 10 - 25 mg/kg/day equally divided q 8 - 12 hrs (not to exceed 250 mg/injection)
		> 40 kg: 250 - 300 mg/day equally divided q 8 - 12 hrs
		IV:
		Older infants and children: 10 - 20 mg/kg/day equally divided q 12 hrs
		> 40 kg: 250 - 500 mg/dose q 6 - 12 hrs depending on severity of illness
			CNS: Dizziness, vertigo, ataxia, drowsiness, fatigue, increased intracranial pressure and bulging fontanel in infants
			CV: Pericarditis
			GI: Nausea, vomiting, diarrhea, epigastric distress, stomatitis, glossitis, dysphagia, black hair tongue, esophageal ulceration, oral candidiasis, pseudomembranous colitis, staphylococcal enterocolitis
			Hepatic: Hepatotoxicity
			GU: Vaginal candidiasis, increased BUN
			Hemic: Leukocytosis, neutropenia, eosinophilia
			Other: Local: IM pain and induration; IV thrombophlebitis, skeletal retardation and tooth staining in young children
				Drugs: Chelates with divalent or trivalent cations (drugs containing aluminum, calcium, magnesium, iron, zinc); may potentiate oral anticoagulants; fatal toxicity if used with methoxyflurane anesthesia.
				
				Food: None
					• Obtain baseline renal, hepatic, and hematologic studies if long term therapy.
					• Obtain culture and sensitivity prior to starting medication.
					• Check expiration date - outdated medication may cause nephrotoxicity.
					• Give on empty stomach as food decreases absorption by 50%.
					• May cause esophageal irritation so do not administer at bedtime to children with reflux and follow with plenty of water.
					• Note preparation - IM and IV preparations not interchangeable !
					• Begin po form as soon as possible as IV causes thrombophlebitis.
					• Patient/parent education:
					  - Finish all medication as prescribed.
					  - Observe for side effects such as superinfection.
					  - Teach proper administration technique.
					  - Protect child from sun.

Name	Uses	Route and Dose	Adverse Reactions/ Side Effects	Drug or Food Interactions	Nursing Considerations
Generic: Ticarcillin **Trade:** Ticar Ticarcipen	Penicillin used to treat infections of the GU and respiratory tracts, intraabdominal, skin and soft tissue infections, and septicemia and meningitis.	**IV:** **Neonates < 2 kg:** ≤ **7 days:** 150 mg/kg/day equally divided q 8h > **7 days:** 225 mg/kg/day equally divided q 8h **Neonates > 2 kg:** ≤ **7 days:** 225 mg/kg/day equally divided q 8h > **7 days:** 300 mg/kg/day equally divided q 8h **Children and adults:** 200 - 300 mg/kg/day equally divided q 4 - 6h	**CNS:** Neuromuscular irritability, seizures with high serum levels **GI:** Nausea, vomiting, abnormal taste, flatulence, loose stools, diarrhea **Hepatic:** Elevation of SGOT, SGPT, LDH, alkaline phosphatase, bilirubin **Hemic:** Anemia, eosinophilia, thrombocytopenia, leukopenia, neutropenia, abnormal PTT and clotting time (with high doses) **Other:** Skin rashes, pruritus, urticaria, drug fever, hypernatremia, hypokalemia **Local:** IV administration - pain, venous irritation, phlebitis; IM administration - pain induration	**Drugs:** Increased risk of bleeding with anticoagulants; decreased effects with erythromycin, tetracycline, and chloromycetin; decreased serum levels with probenecid. **Foods:** None	* Assess for previous allergy to this drug, penicillins, cephalosporins, other drugs, and history of other allergies. * Obtain culture and sensitivity prior to starting medication. * Obtain baseline renal, hepatic, hematologic studies and potassium levels if therapy is to be long-term. * Although slow intermittent IV infusion preferred, may give IV push if diluted to 200 mg/ml and given over 10 minutes. * Monitor for hypersensitivity (especially in first 20 minutes following first administration). * Monitor potassium and sodium levels as well as renal and hepatic function. * Monitor platelets and PTT if on long term therapy. * Maintain appropriate fluid levels for weight.

Name	Uses	Route and Dose	Adverse Reactions/ Side Effects	Drug or Food Interactions	Nursing Considerations
Generic: Tobramycin **Trade:** Tobrex	Aminoglycoside used to treat gram + and - bacteria causing infections of bone, skin, urinary tract, gastrointestinal tract, and neonatal and bacterial septicemias.	**IM,IV:** **Neonates ≤ 7 days:** **< 28 weeks:** 2.5 mg/kg q 24h **28 - 34 weeks:** 2.5 mg/kg q 18h **Term:** 2.5 mg/kg q 12h **Neonates > 7 days:** **< 28 weeks:** 2.5 mg/kg q 18h **28 - 34 weeks:** 2.5 mg/kg q 12h **Infants, 7 days - 1 year:** 2.5 mg/kg q 8h **> 1 year:** 2 - 2.5 mg/kg q 8h **Children:** 7.5 mg/kg/day q equally divided q 8h	**CNS:** Neurotoxicity, neuromuscular blockade, numbness, tingling, muscle twitching and weakness, respiratory depression, lethargy, headache **GI:** Nausea, vomiting, loss of appetite **Hepatic:** Increased bilirubin, SGOT, SGPT, hepatomegaly, hepatic necrosis **GU:** Nephrotoxicity, increased BUN and serum creatinine, decreased urine specific gravity, renal failure **Skin:** Rash, burning, edema **Hemic:** Agranulocytosis, anemia, leukopenia, eosinophilia, thrombocytopenia **Sensory:** Ototoxicity, hearing loss due to damage to eighth cranial nerve, cochlear damage indicated by high frequency hearing loss	**Drugs:** Increased chance of ototoxicity and nephrotoxicity if used concurrently with amphotericin B, salicylates, parenteral bacitracin, antineoplastics, vancomycin; masked symptoms of ototoxicity if used with dimenhydrinate; increased chance of ototoxicity if used with other aminoglycosides; increased respiratory depressant effects of opioids and analgesics, inactivated by parenteral carbenicillin and ticarcillin. **Foods:** None	• Obtain culture and sensitivity prior to starting medication. • Obtain baseline weights, BUN and creatinine, and hearing tests. • Do not infuse in less than 20 minutes. • Monitor for signs of respiratory depression during IV infusion. • Do not give IV push or rapid infusion. • Monitor blood levels of medication. • Observe for adverse reactions/side effects. • Discontinue therapy if no improvement in 3 - 5 days. • Monitor hearing function. • Patient/parent education: - Finish all medication. - Observe for side effects, including hearing loss. - Teach proper administration technique. - If no improvement in 3 - 5 days, notify MD. - If using ointment for ocular infection, do not share towels, wash cloths, pillow cases, make-up, or the medication with others. - Do not wear contact lens if using eye medication.

Name	Uses	Route and Dose	Adverse Reactions/ Side Effects	Drug or Food Interactions	Nursing Considerations

Generic: Vancomycin
 	
Trade: Vancocin
	Effective against gram + bacterial infections. Not effective against gram - infections.	**PO:** 40 mg/kg/day equally divided q 6 - 8h (max.dose = 2 g/day)
		
		IV:
		Neonates ≤ 7 days:
		< 1000 gm: 10 mg/kg q 24h
		1000 - 2000 gm: 10 mg/kg q 18h
		> 2000 gm: 10 mg/kg q 12h
		
		Neonates > 7 days:
		< 1000 gm: 10 mg/kg q 18h
		1000 - 2000 gm: 10 mg/kg q 12h
		> 2000 gm: 10 mg/kg q 8h
		
		Older infants and children:
		CNS infection: 45 mg/kg/day q 8h
		Other infections: 30 mg/kg/day q 8h
			CV: Hypotension with rapid infusion, wheezing, dyspnea **GI:** Nausea **GU:** Transient elevations in BUN and serum creatinine, hyaline and granular casts, albumin in urine, nephrotoxicity, fatal uremia **Hemic:** Leukopenia, eosinophilia, neutropenia **Sensory:** Ototoxicity, permanent deafness due to eighth cranial nerve damage, tinnitus **Other:** Tissue necrosis, pain, thrombophlebitis, anaphylaxis, vascular collapse with hypersensitivity	**Drugs:** Causes erythema and histamine-like flushing when used with anesthetic agents; increased ototoxicity and nephrotoxicity if used with other drugs that have this side effect.
				
				Foods: None
					• Obtain culture and sensitivity prior to starting medication.
					• Obtain renal function tests, BUN and creatinine, hematological tests and hearing tests.
					• Infuse over 60 minutes.
					• Monitor for signs of respiratory depression during IV infusion.
					• Assure patency of IV catheter prior to IV infusion as extravasation causes tissue necrosis .
					• Do not give IM, IV push, or rapid infusion.
					• Do not mix with other drugs.
					• Monitor blood levels of medication.
					• Observe for adverse reactions/side effects, especially tinnitus.
					• Monitor hearing function.
					• Patient/parent education:
					  - Finish all medication.
					  - Observe for side effects, including hearing loss .
					  - Maintain good oral hygiene.
					  - Do not take OTC medications without consulting MD.

Table 3. ANTIFUNGALS

Name	Uses	Route and Dose	Adverse Reactions/ Side Effects	Drug or Food Interactions	Nursing Considerations
Generic: Amphotericin B **Trade:** Fungizone	Antifungal used to treat serious and potentially fatal fungal infections.	**Topical:** Apply BID - QID **IV:** (Mix with D₅W to a concentration of 0.1 mg/ml and pH > 4.2) **Test dose:** 0.1 mg/kg/day up to a max. of 1 mg/dose **Initial dose:** 0.25 mg/kg/day and increase to 1 mg/kg/day as tolerated by increments of 0.123 - 0.25 mg/kg/day or QOD **Max. dose:** 1.5 mg/kg/day Alternate dosing: 1.5 mg/kg/day QOD	**CNS:** Headache, peripheral nerve pain, paresthesia, vision changes, arachnoiditis **GI:** Anorexia, weight loss, dyspepsia, epigastric pain, nausea, vomiting **GU:** Hypokalemia (80% of patients), hyposthenuria, azotemia, renal tubular acido-sis, nephrocalcinosis, permanent renal impairment, anuria, oliguria **Hemic:** Leukopenia, eosinophilia, thrombocytopenia, agranulocytosis, reversible normocytic, normochromic anemia **Skin:** Lotion - pruritus, exacerbation of preexisting candidal lesions; cream - drying effect, erythema, burning contact dermatitis **Musculoskeletal:** Muscle weakness, muscle and joint pain **Other:** Febrile reaction to IV administration, fever and chills 1 - 2 hrs after starting IV infusion, pain at infusion site, phlebitis, thrombophlebitis	**Drugs:** Increased incidence of nephrotoxicity when given with other drugs with the same side effect; enhanced potassium loss if given with corticosteroids, cardiac glycosides, or skeletal muscle relaxants; use with caution with antineoplastic drugs. **Foods:** None	• Obtain positive identification of organism prior to starting treatment with this drug. • Obtain baseline BUN, serum creatinine, liver function tests, hematologic tests, and weight. • Do not use reconstituted medication if not clear of precipitate and/or foreign matter. • Do not mix with other medications. • Infuse very slowly (usually over 6 hours). • Protect infusion from light. • Obtain full sets of vital signs (including temperature) q 30 minutes during infusion. • Monitor for cardiovascular collapse. • Assess I & O, weight, potassium, magnesium, BUN, serum creatinine, bilirubin, alkaline phosphatase, and SGOT QD until routine dose established then q week. • Obtain weekly CBC. • Monitor for signs of hypokalemia. • Patient/parent education: - Teach proper application of topical medications. - If no improvement noted in 2 weeks, contact MD. - Treatment may last several months. - May stain clothing. - Remove lotion from hands with soap and warm water. - Remove ointment from hands with cleaning fluid. - Do not apply OTC medications over infected area without consulting MD.

Name	Uses	Route and Dose	Adverse Reactions/ Side Effects	Drug or Food Interactions	Nursing Considerations

Generic: Griseofulvin
 	
Trade: Fulvicin-U/F
	Antifungal	**PO:**
		> 2 years: 15 - 20 mg/kg/day
			CNS: Headache (early in therapy), fatigue, dizziness, insomnia
			GI: Nausea, vomiting, epigastric distress, polydipsia, flatulence, diarrhea, oral thrush
			Skin: Photosensitivity, urticaria, rashes, angioedema, serumlike sickness
			Hemic: Leukopenia
			Other: Estrogenlike effects, lupus erythematosus or lupuslike syndromes
				Drugs: Flushing and tachycardia with concurrent ingestion of alcohol; decreased drug concentrations with phenobarbital; decrease in PTT if given with warfarin; breakthrough bleeding with oral contraceptives
				
				Food: Enhanced absorption if given with high fat diet
					• Obtain positive identification of organism prior to starting treatment with this drug.
					• Obtain CBC, renal and hepatic tests prior to long term therapy.
					• Give with food to decrease GI distress.
					• Increase absorption by giving with high-fat meal.
					• Monitor for headache.
					• Observe for side effects.
					• Continue treatment until 2 - 3 negative weekly cultures and replacement of infected skin, hair, and/or nails.
					• Patient/parent education:
					  - Therapy requires close monitoring by MD.
					  - Therapy lasts between 4 weeks and several months.
					  - Avoid exposure to sun.

Name	Uses	Route and Dose	Adverse Reactions/ Side Effects	Drug or Food Interactions	Nursing Considerations
Generic: Miconazole **Trade:** Monistat Micatin	Antifungal	**IV:** **> 1 yr.:** 15 - 40 mg/kg/day equally divided q 8h (max. dose = 15 mg/kg/dose) **Topical:** Apply BID x 2 - 4 weeks **Intrathecal:** 20 mg/dose q 1 - 2 days **Vaginal:** 1 applicatorful q HS x 7 days	**CNS:** Dizziness, drowsiness, headache, IT administration - arachnoiditis, transient saddle numbness, <u>12th cranial nerve palsy, mild third ventricular hemorrhage</u> **GI:** Nausea, vomiting, anorexia **Skin:** Pruritus (IV), irritation, burning, maceration (topical) **Hemic:** Transient decrease in hematocrit, normocytic or microcytic anemia, <u>thrombocytopenia</u> **Other:** Fever, chills, flushing, hyperlipidemia, serum triglycerides, hyponatremia **Local:** Phlebitis	**Drugs:** Altered metabolism if given with cyclosporine, phenytoin, rifampin; antagonized if used with amphotericin B; enhanced anticoagulant effects if used with coumarin drugs. **Foods:** None	• Obtain positive identification of organism prior to starting treatment with this drug. • Obtain baseline hct, hgb, serum electrolytes, and lipids. • Discard IV solution if dark in color. • Infuse over 30 - 60 minutes. • Do not mix with other drugs. • Do not use vaginal suppositories with latex diaphragms or condoms. • Monitor for cardiac arrhythmias during infusion. • Monitor for phlebitis. • Observe for side effects. • Monitor hct, hgb, serum electrolytes, and lipids. • Patient/parent education: - Teach proper application of topical forms. - Therapy usually lasts between 6 - 12 weeks. - If no improvement in 2 weeks, contact MD. - Wear panty liner to prevent staining of underwear. - Do not apply other OTC topical medications without consulting MD.

Name	Uses	Route and Dose	Adverse Reactions/ Side Effects	Drug or Food Interactions	Nursing Considerations
Generic: Nystatin **Trade:** Mycostatin	Antifungal	**PO:** **Premature Infants, neonates:** 100,000 U QID **Children:** 400,000 - 600,000 U QID **Topical:** Apply sufficient amount to cover affected area QD **Vaginal:** 1 suppository or applicatorful q HS x 7 days	**GI:** Transient nausea, vomiting, diarrhea **Skin:** Rare topical irritation usually a reaction to preservatives	**Drugs:** None noted. **Foods:** None	• Obtain positive identification of organism but may start therapy prior to identification. • Assist patient in having good oral hygiene. • Do not give fluids for 30 minutes following administration. • If child is old enough, have him swish medication in for as long as possible before swallowing. • Provide good oral hygiene 30 minutes following administration (many solutions contain up to 50% sucrose). • Wear gloves when applying topically. • If using powder, do not inhale particles. • Do not cover areas with occlusive dressings. • Give vaginal medication during menstruation. • If skin irritation occurs, discontinue and notify MD. • Patient/parent education: - Teach proper application of topical forms. - Continue medication for full course of therapy as prescribed by MD. - Teach good oral hygiene to prevent reinfection. - Wear panty liner to prevent staining of underwear. - Do not apply other OTC topical medications without consulting MD. - Discard or disinfect toothbrush. - Children should not share towels or clothes during treatment.

Table 4. ANTIVIRALS

Name	Uses	Route and Dose	Adverse Reactions/ Side Effects	Drug or Food Interactions	Nursing Considerations
Generic: Ribavirin **Trade:** Virazole	Antiviral used to treat severe lower respiratory infections caused by respiratory syncytial virus (RSV).	**Inhalation:** 190 mcg/L in mist by Viratek small-particle aerosol generator (SPAG-2) per oxygen hood or face mask at a rate of 12.5 - L mist per minute over 12 - 18 h for a minimum of 3 days and a maximum of 7 days.	**CV:** Hypotension, <u>cardiac arrest</u> **Resp:** Worsening of respiratory function, <u>dyspnea, bacterial pneumonia, pneumothorax,</u> ventilator dependence **Skin:** Rash **Hemic:** Reticulocytosis, anemia **Sensory:** Erythema of eyelids, conjunctivitis	**Drugs:** Studies are incomplete although it appears that the antiviral activity of zidovudine against HIV may be antagonized and the antiviral activity of other agents may be enhanced. **Foods:** None	• Treatment may be started prior to obtaining culture but should not continue for more than 24 hrs before positive confirmation of RSV infection. • Do not use with mild or moderate infections. • Most effective in the first 3 days of infection. • Drug is teratogenic in animal studies; question family and visitors about possible pregnancy. • Pregnant staff members should not have prolonged contact with mist. • Staff should not wear soft contact lens while caring for child (causes crystallization of contacts). • Do not administer with any other aerosol medications. • Assess respiratory function carefully. • Informed consent is required by the FDA prior to administering to any child on a ventilator. • Patient/parent education: - Give information about disease process. - Provide information on isolation procedures. - Provide information about drug therapy.

Name	Uses	Route and Dose	Adverse Reactions/ Side Effects	Drug or Food Interactions	Nursing Considerations
Generic: Acyclovir **Trade:** Zorivax	Antiviral used to treat cytomegalovirus and herpes simplex infections and varicella zoster infections in immunocompromised children.	**PO:** **Genital HSV:** 200 mg x 5 doses/day for 5 days **IV:** **Neonates:** 30 mg/kg/day equally divided q 8h **Children < 12 years:** 750 mg/m^2/day equally divided q 8h **Children > 5 years:** 5 mg/kg equally divided q 8h	**CNS:** Headache, dizziness, fatigue, insomnia, irritability, depression, IV administration - lethargy, obtundation, tremors, confusion, hallucinations, agitation, seizures, coma **CV:** Hypotension, palpitations **GI:** Nausea, vomiting, diarrhea **Hepatic:** Transient rise in SGOT, SGPT, alkaline phosphatase **GU:** Hematuria, transient rise in serum creatinine **Skin:** Rash, urticaria, acne, accelerated hair loss **Hemic:** Thrombocytosis, thrombocytopenia, leukopenia, lymphopenia **Musculoskeletal:** Arthralgia, pars planitis, muscle cramps, leg pain **Other:** Fever, sore throat, lymphadenopathy, superficial thrombophlebitis	**Drugs:** Half-life and renal clearance increased if given with probenecid; use cautiously with children who have had previous interferon or cytotoxic induced neurologic reactions; cautious use in children receiving intrathecal methotrexate. **Foods:** None	• Record appearance and number of lesions. • Confirm diagnosis with culture of lesions. • Give drug at first sign of infection (tingling, burning, itching, or pain). • Do not give drug SC, IM, ID, or ophthalmically. • Do not give IV push. • Wear gloves when applying topical drug (HS virus has been reported to have survived 88 hrs on inanimate objects). • Provide adequate hydration during and after IV administration. • Monitor for CNS symptoms. • Assess urinary function (I & O, renal function studies). • Avoid extravasation. • Patient/parent education: - Provide information on application of drug to avoid spread of disease. - Teach good handwashing technique. - Children should have separate wash cloths and towels and should not share clothing. - Provide information/education on how the disease is spread, S & S of infection, prevention of transmission to others.

Table 5. CNS MEDICATIONS

Name	Uses	Route and Dose	Adverse Reactions/ Side Effects	Drug or Food Interactions	Nursing Considerations
Generic: Caffeine **Trade:** Caffedrine	CNS stimulant used to treat neonatal apnea.	**SC,IM,IV: CNS stimulation:** 8 mg/kg not to exceed 500 mg **PO,IM,IV: Neonatal apnea:** 5 - 10 mg/kg as loading dose followed by 1 - 5 mg/kg/day (not to exceed 12 mg/kg/ day in two doses)	**CNS:** Insomnia, restlessness, nervousness, deli-rium, dizziness, tremors, headache, confusion, irrita-bility, seizures, anxiety, tinnitus **CV:** Increased pulse, arrhythmia **GI:** Abdominal distention and vomiting in neonates, nausea, diarrhea, gastric irritation **GU:** Bacteriuria, nephritis, frequency **Other:** Kernicterus in neonates	**Drugs:** Increased inotropic effects of beta blockers; increased metabolism of barbiturates; increased side effects of other xanthines (i.e., aminophylline); inhibits calcium absorption; increased half-life if given with disulfiram. **Foods:** None	• Take baseline vital signs. • Do not use during respiratory and cardiac failure. • Use only citrated injection for neona- tal apnea (other preparations may cause kernicterus). • Give slowly. • Monitor vital signs during administration. • Draw blood levels 24 hrs following initial dose and then 1 - 2 x week.

Name	Uses	Dose and Route	Adverse Reactions/ Side Effects	Drug or Food Interactions	Nursing Considerations

Generic: Carbamazepine
 	
Trade: Tegretol
	Anticonvulsant used to treat psychomotor, clonic-tonic, and mixed seizures. Also provides pain relief from trigeminal neuralgia. Also used without FDA approval to treat pain and symptoms of multiple sclerosis, hemifacial spasm, dystonia, and antidiuretic effects in diabetes insipidus.	**PO:**
		< 6 yrs: 5 mg/kg/day increasing to 10 mg/kg/day in 5 - 7 days prn and then to 20 mg/kg/day in 5 - 7 days prn.
		6 - 12 yrs: 100 mg BID increasing by 100 mg/day in weekly intervals prn. Doses should not > 1 g/day and should be given TID or QID if daily dose > 200 mg. Usual maintenance dose is 400 - 800 mg/day.
		> 12 yrs: 200 mg BID increasing by up to 200 mg/day prn in weekly intervals. Doses should not > 1 g/day for patients 13 - 15 yrs and 1.2 g/day for > 15 yrs. Doses should be given TID or QID if daily dose > 400 mg. Usual maintenance dose is 800 - 1200 mg/day.
			CNS: Ataxia and dizziness (plasma levels ≤ 10 mg/ml), nystagmus (plasma levels . 4 mg/ml), drowsiness, vertigo, diplopia, speech changes, involuntary movements; behavior changes, weakness, headache, depression, trembling, hallucinations
			CV: CHF, hypertension, hypotension, thrombophlebitis, arrhythmia, chest pain, changes in heart rate
			GI: Nausea, vomiting, diarrhea, GI pain, constipation, dry mouth, sore throat, mouth ulcers
			Resp: Dyspnea, pneumonia
			Hepatic: Jaundice, hepatitis, abnormal liver function tests
			GU: Frequency, retention, oliguria, renal failure, SIADH
			Skin: Rash, urticaria, pigmentation changes (especially with light exposure), alopecia, worsening of lupus erythematosus
			Hemic: Aplastic anemia, leukopenia, eosinophilia, thrombocytopenia, agranulocytosis, leukocytosis
			Other: Fever, aching joints, muscle cramps, ocular changes
				Drugs: Decreased serum concentrations if used with phenytoin, phenobarbital, doxycycline, and warfarin; breakthrough bleeding with oral contraceptives; increased serum levels when used with verapamil or erythromycin; do not give with monoamine oxidase inhibitors.
				
				Foods: None
					* Take baseline CBC, platelet, reticulocyte, iron studies, liver function tests, BUN, ECG, UA, EEG, and eye studies.
					* This medication is used only with children who have had serious side effects or no change in seizure activity when utilizing other anticonvulsant medications.
					* Should not be used in children suffering from mixed seizure disorders as it worsens seizure activity.
					* Give with food to increase absorption.
					* Monitor CBC, platelets, reticulocytes, and iron counts q week x 3 months and then monthly. Drug should be dc'd if RBC is < 4 million/mm³, hct < 32%, hgb < 11 g/dl, WBC < 4000/mm³, reticulocyte < 20,000/mm³, platelet count < 100,000/ mm³, or serum iron is > 150 mcg/dl.
					* Regularly monitor liver function tests, renal studies (including BUN and UA), serum electrolytes, and eye studies.
					* Patient/parent education:
					  - Take drug only as directed.
					  - Do not operate machinery or drive a car.
					  - Do not stop medication suddenly.
					  - Avoid sunlight exposure.
					  - Notify MD immediately if bleeding, bruising, fever, sore throat or fatigue occur.
					  - See MD regularly.
					  - Wear bracelet stating that patient suffers from seizures and takes anticonvulsant medication.

Name	Uses	Route and Dose	Adverse Reactions/ Side Effects	Drug or Food Interactions	Nursing Considerations
Generic: Clonazepan **Trade:** Clonapin	Anticonvulsant used in absence, akinetic, and myoclonic seizures. Also used without FDA approval to treat tonic-clonic, psychomotor, and infantile spasm seizures.	**PO:** **< 10 yrs or 30 kg:** 0.01 - 0.03 mg/kg/day initially in 2 - 3 doses (not to exceed 0.05 mg/kg/day in 2 - 3 doses); dosage is increased no more than 0.5 mg q 3 days and maintenance dose should not exceed 0.2 mg/kg/day **Older children:** 1.5 mg/day initially with dosage increased 0.5 - 1.0 mg q 3 days and maintenance should not exceed 20 mg/day.	**CNS:** Sedation, drowsiness, ataxia, behavior changes especially in those with brain damage, mental retardation, or mental illness, aggression, irritability, hyperactivity, confusion, depression, headache, dizziness, tremor, vertigo, insomnia **CV:** Palpitation **GI:** Constipation, gastritis, anorexia, nausea, dry mouth, thirst, sore gums **Resp:** Increased secretions, dyspnea, difficulty swallowing **Hepatic:** Hepatomegaly, liver enzyme changes **GU:** Dysuria, enuresis, retention, nocturia **Skin:** Hirsutism or hair loss, rash **Hemic:** Anemia, leukopenia, thrombocytopenia, eosinophilia **Other:** Fever, dehydration, lymphadenopathy	**Drugs:** Increased depressant effects if used with CNS depressants; increases serum phenytoin levels; increased serum levels when used with cimetidine or disulfiram; decreased serum levels of both if used with carbamazepine. **Foods:** None	• Take baseline weight, height, liver function studies, and CBC. • Record seizure activity. • Tolerance may develop as soon as 3 months, necessitating changes in drug regime. • Measure height and weight regularly. • Monitor liver function studies and CBC periodically. • Monitor behavior changes. • Patient/parent education: - Take drug only as directed. - Do not operate machinery or drive a car. - Do not stop medication suddenly. - Report continuing symptoms of drowsiness and ataxia (these should decrease as therapy continues). - Avoid alcohol, CNS depressants, and other medications unless prescribed by MD. - Wear bracelet stating that patient suffers from seizures and takes anticonvulsant medication.

Name	Uses	Dose and Route	Adverse Reactions/ Side Effects	Drug or Food Interactions	Nursing Considerations
Generic: Pentobarbital **Trade:** Nembutal	Barbiturate used as a hypnotic for short term treatment of insomnia, as treatment for status epilepticus and severe seizures, and as an adjunct to anesthesia.	**PO:** **Sedation:** 2 - 6 mg/kg/day (max. dose = 100 mg/day) **Preoperative Medication:** < 10 yrs: 5 mg/kg; 10 - 12 yrs: 100 mg **IM:** **Hypnosis:** 2 - 6 mg/kg (max. dose = 100 mg) **IV:** **Initial dose:** 50 mg **PR:** **Hypnosis:** 2 mo. - 1 yr: 30 mg; 1 - 4 yrs: 30 - 60 mg; 5 - 12 yrs: 60 mg; 12 - 14 yrs: 60 - 120 mg **Sedation:** 2 - 6 mg/kg/day (max. dose = 100 mg/day)	**CNS:** Drowsiness, lethargy, headache, vertigo, mental depression, impaired motor skills **CV:** Vasodilation, hypotension **GI:** Nausea, vomiting, diarrhea, constipation **Resp:** Respiratory depression, apnea, bronchospasm, laryngospasm, especially with rapid IV infusion **Hepatic:** Hepatitis, jaundice **Skin:** Thrombophlebitis at IV site, hypersensitivity reaction with skin rash, urticaria, dermatitis, systemic lupus erythematosus	**Drugs:** Potentiates other CNS depressants; decreased GI absorption of dicumarol; decreased levels of corticosteroids; decreased levels of griseofulvin; decreased half-life of doxycycline; decreased effectiveness of birth control pills; increased respiratory depressant effects with other drugs having this effect. **Food:** None	• Take baseline vital signs and assess for allergy to barbiturates and respiratory disease. • Take po medications on empty stomach. • Check injectable preparations for precipitate. • Incompatible with many drugs - do not mix when giving IV. • Take vital signs frequently during administration. • Do not use for longer than 2 weeks to treat insomnia. • Monitor for bruising, fever, sore throat, bleeding and discontinue drug if these are present. • Observe for skin reactions. These are potentially fatal and drug should be discontinued if they are noted. • Patient/parent education: - Take drug only as directed. - Do not operate machinery or drive a car. - Report signs of fever, sore throat, bleeding, bruising, or skin reaction. - Avoid alcohol, CNS depressants, and other medications unless prescribed by MD. - Drug may be habit forming and long-term use requires a slow withdrawal.

Name	Uses	Dose and Route	Adverse Reactions/ Side Effects	Drug or Food Interactions	Nursing Considerations
Generic: Phenobarbital **Trade:** Luminal	Anticonvulsant, barbiturate used for all types of seizures except absence. Also used as hypnotic and sedative.	**PO:** **Seizures:** 3 - 5 mg/kg/day **Febrile seizures:** 3 - 4 mg/kg/day **Sedation:** 6 mg/kg/day **Preoperative sedation:** 1 - 3 mg/kg **IM:** **Preoperative sedation:** 16 - 100 mg 60 - 90 minutes before surgery **IV:** **Status Epilepticus:** 15 - 20 mg/kg over 10 - 15 minutes	**CNS:** Drowsiness, ataxia, irritability, headache, paradoxical excitement, hyperactivity, sleep disturbance, impaired memory, school difficulties **GI:** Nausea, vomiting **Hepatic:** Hepatitis, jaundice **GU:** Renal damage **Skin:** Rash, dermatitis **Hemic:** Lowered RBC levels, bone marrow suppression **Metabolic:** Hypocalcemia	**Drugs:** Possibly increases or decreases phenytoin levels; decreases serum levels of corticosteroids, tricyclic antidepressants, griseofulvin, doxycycline, and digoxin; increases depressant effects of alcohol and other CNS depressants. **Food:** None	• Take baseline CBC, liver function tests, UA. • Assess history of child's school performance. • May mix po forms with food. • Inject IM doses deep into large muscle - inadvertent SC injection may cause tissue necrosis. • May mix with most IV solutions. • Use reconstituted solution within 30 minutes and do not use if precipitate noted. • Incompatible with many drugs - do not mix for administration. • IV administration not to exceed 2 mg/kg/min or 30 mg/min. • Monitor level of consciousness. • Monitor vital signs, CBC, liver and renal function tests if on long-term therapy. • Monitor school performance if on longterm therapy. • Observe for signs of hypocalcemia. • Patient/parent education: - Take drug only as directed. - Do not d/c medication, alter dose or change forms without consulting MD. - Do not take other drugs or alcohol with this medication. - Report increasing dizziness, lethargy, ataxia, changes in school performance to MD.

Name	Uses	Dose and Route	Adverse Reactions/ Side Effects	Drug or Food Interactions	Nursing Considerations
Generic: Phenytoin **Trade:** Dilantin	Anticonvulsant used for tonic-clonic and partial seizures as well as seizures with nonepilepsy cause.	**PO:** **Seizures:** 5 mg/kg in 2 - 3 doses initially adjusted prn but not to exceed 300 mg/day. Usual maintenance dose is 4 - 8 mg/kg/day or 200 mg/day. Loading dose may be used to achieve serum levels more quickly. **IM:** Use only temporarily if patient unable to tolerate po dose. To establish IM dose, take usual po dose and divide in half. After returning to po dose, maintain half dose for 1 week due to chance of slow release of IM drug. **IV:** **Status Epilepticus:** 10 - 15 mg/kg but not to exceed 20 mg/kg/day	**CNS:** Confusion, drowsiness during early therapy, dizziness, headache; nystagmus, diplopia and ataxia indicate intoxication **CV:** Cardiovascular arrest, hypotension with IV use **GI:** Nausea, vomiting, anorexia, decreased sense of taste, weight loss **Skin:** Pain and necrosis at injection site, rash or severe dermatitis with fever, lupus erythematosus, Stevens-Johnson syndrome, hirsutism (particularly in females) **Hemic:** Thrombocytopenia, leukopenia, granulocytopenia, pancytopenia, anemia **Endocrine:** Hyperglycemia **Other:** Lymphadenopathy, hypertrichosis, osteomalacia, gingival hyperplasia	**Drugs:** Serum levels decreased by CNS depressants, antacids, barbiturates, folic acid, rifampin, valproic acid (may also increase levels); increased sedation with primidone; may decrease serum digoxin levels; increased levels with disulfiram. **Foods:** May interfere with Vitamin D absorption and folic acid metabolism.	• Take baseline CBC, liver function tests, UA. • Assess vital signs before starting IV. • Assess previous skin reactions to phenytoin administration. • Note type of phenytoin used - chewable tabs and suspension are phenytoin sodium and contain less phenytoin. Bioavailability depends on brand of phenytoin used. • PO forms should be given with food to decrease gastric distress. • Give IM only if PO cannot be tolerated. • IV solution should be clear or slightly yellow - do not use if any precipitate noted. • Give IV no faster than 0.5 - 1.5 mg/kg/min. • Do not mix with other medications. • Clear line with normal saline flush before and after IV injection. • Monitor CBC, liver functions, and UA if on long-term therapy. • Monitor serum drug levels. • Patient/parent education: - Take drug only as directed. - Do not d/c medication, alter dose or change forms or brands without consulting MD. - Do not take other drugs or alcohol. - Teach family emergency care for seizures and to report all seizure activity. - Drug can alter alertness - avoid driving and alter activities accordingly. - Teach oral hygiene as soon as teeth erupt. - Report classroom performance.

Name	Uses	Dose and Route	Adverse Reactions/ Side Effects	Drug or Food Interactions	Nursing Considerations

Generic: Valproic acid
 	
Trade: Depakene, Depakote
	Used alone or combined with other CNS medications for simple and complex absence (petit mal) seizures. Also used without FDA approval for other types of seizures.	**PO:** 15 mg/kg/day initially. May be increased by 5 - 10 mg/kg/day PRN. Should not exceed 60 mg/kg/day. Usually given in 2 divided doses.	**CNS:** Drowsiness, headache, tremor, anxiety, confusion, paresthesia, dizziness, incoordination; hyperactivity and behavior changes more common in children
			GI: Nausea, vomiting, indigestion (common); hypersalivation, anorexia, weight loss, diarrhea, constipation, cramps
			Hepatic: Hepatotoxicity with increased liver enzymes, most common in children < 2 yrs who are receiving other drugs, have metabolic disease or mental retardation
			GU: Enuresis
			Skin: Rash, hair loss or changes, facial swelling
			Hemic: Decreased platelet aggregation and prolonged bleeding time; bruising, thrombocytopenia, leukopenia, eosinophilia, anemia, decreased fibrinogen
				Drugs: Increased CNS depression if used with other CNS depressants; increases phenobarbital and primidone levels; not recommended with clonazepam due to possible seizure activity; may alter binding and action of phenytoin; potentiates MAO inhibitors and antidepressants; use cautiously with anticoagulants; may increases folic acid needs; increased risk of hepatotoxicity in young children taking other anticonvulsants or hepatotoxic medications.
				
				Foods: None
					• Obtain baseline renal and liver function tests, CBC, coagulation tests, and serum ammonia.
					• Do not give medication if abnormal liver function or coagulation tests or hyperammonia.
					• Monitor liver function tests frequently - especially in first 6 months when risk of hepatotoxicity is greatest.
					• Coagulation studies should be monitored periodically and prior to any surgical procedures.
					• Give with food to decrease gastric distress.
					• Patient/parent education:
					  - Take drug only as directed.
					  - Do not change dosage of medication.
					  - Return for scheduled follow up visits.
					  - Avoid OTC medications and alcohol.
					  - Avoid driving and adjust activities due to altered mental alertness.
					  - Notify MD's of use of this medication prior to having surgery or dental work.
					  - Child should wear identification bracelet stating history of seizure activity and use of valproic acid.

Table 6. BROCHODILATORS/PULMONARY MEDICATIONS

Name	Uses	Route and Dose	Adverse Reactions/ Side Effects	Drug or Food Interactions	Nursing Considerations
Generic: Acetylcysteine **Trade:** Mucomyst	Mucolytic used to decrease the viscosity of respiratory secretions. Used in treatment of cystic fibrosis, bronchitis, pneumonia, tuberculosis, mucous obstruction atelectasis, and emphysema. Also used to prevent hepatotoxicity in treatment of acetaminophen overdose.	**PO:** **Acetaminophen Overdose:** 140 mg/kg initially followed by 70 mg/kg q 4 hrs x 17 doses **Inhalation:** **Nebulized solution:** 3 - 5 mg of 20% solution or 6 - 10 mg 10% solution TID or QID **Tent or Croupette:** 300 ml of 10 or 20% solution **Intratracheal:** 1 - 2 ml of 10 or 20% solution q 1 - 4h	**CNS:** Drowsiness **GI:** Nausea, vomiting, stomatitis **Resp:** Rhinorrhea, bronchospasm (more common in asthmatics), hemoptysis **Skin:** Urticaria (generalized) **Other:** Fever, chills	**Drugs:** Decreased effectiveness if used with activated charcoal; incompatible with amphotericin B, chlortetracycline HCl, erythromycin lactobionate, oxytetracycline HCl, ampicillin, tetracycline, iodized oil, trypsin, and hydrogen peroxide. **Foods:** None	* Assess baseline respiratory rate and characteristics. * Assess cough for frequency and type and amount and type of secretions. * Draw serum drug levels if acetaminophen ingestion. Treatment may start prior to receiving lab results. Do not delay if ingestion within 24 hours. * Drug most effective if given within 10 - 12 hours of reported ingestion. * May dilute solution for overdose treatment with soft drinks or juice. Use within 1 hour of dilution. * Drug has foul odor (rotten eggs) so administer in container with lid and straw. * If dose vomited within 1 hour, repeat. * If used for overdosage, monitor for other signs of acetaminophen toxicity. * If given via NG or OG tube, dilute prior to administration to prevent irritation or sclerosing of duodenum. * Do not administer via hand held nebulizer due to large particle size. * Use only plastic or glass nebulizer * Do not use heated nebulizer. * Administer with compressed air or oxygen. Administer with caution in patients with CO_2 retention. * Have patient clear airway prior to administration. * Keep continuous nebulizer full to prevent impedance of drug delivery. * Patient/parent education: - Follow teaching plan. - Have regular medical follow up.

Name	Uses	Route and Dose	Adverse Reactions/ Side Effects	Drug or Food Interactions	Nursing Considerations
Generic: Aminophylline **Trade:** Aminophyllin, Somophyllin - DF	Bronchodilator used in treatment of bronchial asthma, chronic bronchitis, and emphysema. Used for apnea of prematurity and bradycardia in neonates.	**PO:** 1 - 9 yrs: 20 mg/kg/day q 6h 9 - 16 yrs: 16 mg/kg/day q 6h > 16 years (adult): 12 mg/kg/day q 6h **IV:** • Neonatal apnea: loading dose = 4 - 6 mg/kg x 1 dose (each 1 mg/kg will raise serum dr level 2 mcg/ml) Maintenance: Preterm infants to 40 weeks postnatal age: 1 mg/kg q 12h Term newborns to 4 weeks postnatal age: 1 - 2 mg/kg q 8h 4 - 8 weeks postnatal age: 1 - 3 mg/kg q 8h • Bronchospasm: loading dose = 6 mg/kg x 1 dose Maintenance: Neonates up to 24 days: 1.25 mg/kg q 12h Neonates > 24 days: 1.9 mg/kg q 12h 1 - 9 yrs: 1 mg/kg/hr 9 - 12 yrs: 0.9 mg/kg/hr 12 - 16 yrs (nonsmoker): 0.6 mg/kg/hr 12 - 16 yrs (smoker): 0.9 mg/kg/hr • Doses must be individualized and based on serum drug levels	**CNS:** Headaches, restlessness, dizziness, irritability, insomnia, muscle twitching, <u>seizures</u> **CV:** Palpitations, <u>sinus tachycardia</u>, extrasystoles, flushing, marked hypotension, <u>circulatory failure, cardiac arrest</u> **GI:** Nausea, vomiting, bitter aftertaste, epigastric pain, anorexia, diarrhea **Resp:** Tachypnea **GU:** Albuminuria **Skin:** Urticaria, exfoliative dermatitis **Other:** Hyperglycemia, SIADH, local redness and pain at IV site	**Drugs:** Serum drug levels increased by phenytoin and barbiturates; decreases effectiveness of lithium and furosemide; beta-adrenergic blockers (especially propranolol and nadolol) may induce broncho-spasms when used concurrently; decreased hepatic clearance with erythromycin, cimetidine, troleandomycin; enhances toxic potential of cardiac glycosides; increased CNS stimulation with adrenergics. **Food:** None	• Assess respiratory status and vital signs. • Weigh patient. • If child is currently taking theophylline, determine when amount and time last dose given. • Withhold dose from neonates with heart rate > 180. • Delayed absorption if given with food, but may administer with meals if GI irritation present. • If IV, <u>do not administer faster than 25 mg/minute</u>. • IV administration rate usually 25 - 30 minutes. • Continuous IV infusion usually given at rate of 0.9 - 1.5 mg/kg/hour. • Do not use continuous infusion for neonates. • Monitor respiratory status. • Monitor serum drug levels frequently and maintain between 10 - 20 mcg/ml. • Check with pharmacist prior to mixing with any drug. • Patient/parent education: - Report any CNS, cardiac, or GI side effects to MD. - Monitor respiratory response. - Maintain hydration and weight. - Do not use any OTC drugs containing ephedrine. - Take as directed and at same time each day to maintain levels.

Name	Uses	Route and Dose	Adverse Reactions/Side Effects	Drugs or Food Interactions	Nursing Considerations
Generic: Epinephrine

Trade: Adrenalin, AsthmaHaler, Breatheasy, Vaponephrin | Adrenergic agonist that causes vasoconstriction, bronchodilation, increased heart rate, and cardiac stimulation. Used to treat cardiac arrest, acute asthma attack or anaphylaxis. Also used as an ophthalmic decongestant. | **IM,IV:** Anaphylaxis: 300 mcg initially and repeated a 15 min 3 - 4 times PRN

SC: Asthma and anaphylaxis: 10 mcg/kg (0.01 ml/kg of 1:1000); not to exceed 500 mcg/dose. Repeat q 15 min x 2 PRN and then give q 4h PRN.

Severe anaphylaxis: 0.1 mg (10 ml of 1:10,000) over 5 - 10 minutes initially followed by continuous IV infusion of 0.1 - 1.5 mcg/kg/min

Bronchodilation with prolonged action: 25 mcg/kg repeated q 6h. Do not exceed 750 mcg in children 30 kg.

Inhalation: > 6 yrs: metered aerosol: 160 - 250 mcg or 1 puff; repeat PRN q 4h

> 6 yrs: hand-bulb nebulizer: 1 - 2 deep inhalations of 1% solution, repeated in 1 - 2 minutes and then q 4h

≥ 4 yrs: Racepinephrine hand-held nebulizer: 2 - 3 puffs of 2.25% solution, repeated in 5 min. PRN. May be given 4 - 6 times/day. | **CNS:** Anxiety, restlessness, dizziness, headache, excitability, weakness, syncope, convulsions, fever, chills **CV:** Tachycardia, palpitations, increased blood pressure, flushing, EKG changes, chest pain, irregular pulse **Resp:** Dyspnea, rebound bronchospasm after withdrawal of inhalation therapy **GI:** Nausea, vomiting **Skin:** Necrosis at injection site with repeated injections; pale cold skin **Sensory:** Blurred vision, enlarged pupils **Other:** Prolonged use can lead to metabolic acidosis | **Drugs:** Additive effects with other sympathomimetics; decreased respiratory and cardiac effects with beta adrenergic blockers; severe hypotension and tachycardia if given with rapid-acting vasodilators; decreased effects with antihypertensives; increased cardiac effects observed if given with some general anesthetics; increased cardiac effects with cardiac clygosides, tricyclic antidepressants, antihistamines, and thyroid medications; monitor EKG if given with digitalis; added CNS effects with other CNS stimulants and xanthines; increased insulin needs with diabetes.

Foods: none | • Baseline vital signs, especially pulse and B/P.
• Evaluate and monitor EKG, blood gases, CVP, and urine output.
• Use 1 mg/ml solution (1:1000) if giving IV.
• Monitor blood glucose in diabetic patients closely.
• Patient/parent education:
  - Teach correct inhalation technique.
  - Do not use solutions that are discolored or have precipitate.
  - Seek medical attention if asthma not improved in 20 minutes following administration .
  - Do not exceed recommended dose.
  - Rinse mouth with water following each dose to prevent dryness. |

Name	Uses	Route and Dose	Adverse Reactions/ Side Effects	Drug or Food Interactions	Nursing Considerations

Generic: Metaproterenol
 	
Trade: Alupent
	Bronchodilator used to manage asthma, prevention of exercise induced asthma, and to enhance therapeutic effects of theophylline	**PO:**
		< 6 yrs: 1.3 - 2.6 mg/kg/day
		6 - 9 yrs (27.3 kg): 10 mg 3 - 4 times/day
		> 9 yrs: 20 mg 3 - 4 times/day
		
		Inhalation: 12 yrs
		Aerosol: 2 - 3 inhalations q 3 - 4h (max. dose 12 inhalations/day)
		Nebulizer solution: 0.2 - 0.3 ml of 5% solution in 2.5 ml of NS or 2.5 ml of 0.6% solution q 4 - 6h
			CNS: Nervousness, tremors, dizziness, headache, drowsiness
			CV: Tachycardia, palpitations, hypertension, cardiac arrest (overdosage)
			GI: Nausea, vomiting, bad taste
			Other: Muscle cramps
				Drugs: Additive effects if used with other sympatho-mimetic amines; broncho-dilation effects antagonized by effects of beta adrenergic blocking agents
				
				Foods: None
					• Assess respiratory status.
					• Obtain baseline heart rate.
					• Do not crush PO tabs. May be ad-ministered with food.
					• Side effects more common with oral forms.
					• Shake inhalation forms well prior to administration.
					• Monitor respiratory response.
					• Maintain hydration.
					• May use po and inhalation forms concurrently.
					• Patient/parent education:
					  - Teach correct inhalation technique.
					  - Do not exceed recommended dose.
					  - Discontinue if paradoxical bronchospasms noted.
					  - Do not use this with any other in-halers.

Name	Uses	Route and Dose	Adverse Reactions/ Side Effects	Drug or Food Interactions	Nursing Considerations
Generic: Terbutaline sulfate **Trade:** Brethine, Brethaire	Bronchial dilator used to treat asthma and emphysema.	**PO:** **> 12 yrs:** 0.05 mg/kg/dose TID (max. dose - 7.5 mg/day) **SC:** **< 12 yrs:** 0.005 - 0.010 mg/kg/dose (max. dose 0.25 mg/dose q 15 - 20 minutes BID) **> 12 yrs:** 3.5 - 5 mcg/kg (max. dose 0.5 mg in 4h) **Inhalation:** 2 inhalations (400 mcg) q 4 - 6h	**CNS:** Nervousness, tremors, dizziness, headache, lethargy, sweating **CV:** Palpitations, tachycardia, dysrhythmia **GI:** Nausea, vomiting **Sensory:** Dry nose, mouth and throat; tinnitus	**Drugs:** Hypertensive crisis with MAO inhibitors; additive effects with other sympathomimetic amines; antagonized bronchodilator effects with beta adrenergic blocking agents. **Foods:** None	• Assess respiratory status. • Obtain baseline heart rate. • Do not crush extended-release tabs. • May crush other tabs and mix with food. • Do not use SC solution if discolored. • **SC doses must be checked with an RN prior to administration. Errors in decimal points may be fatal!** • Monitor cardiac response with SC route. • May repeat SC dose if no improvement in 15 - 30 minutes. • Do not repeat if no improvement after second dose. • Maintain hydration. • Monitor response. • Patient/parent education: - Teach correct inhalation technique. - Do not exceed recommended dose. - Contact MD if symptoms worsen. - Discontinue if paradoxical bronchospasms noted. - Do not use this with any other inhalers.

Name	Uses	Route and Dose	Adverse Reactions/ Side Effects	Drug or Food Interactions	Nursing Considerations
Generic: Theophylline **Trade:** Slo-bid Theo-Dur Slo-Phyllin-12	Bronchodilator used to treat bronchial asthma, chronic bronchitis, and emphysema; apnea of prematurity and bradycardia in preterm infants; bronchial spasms in cystic fibrosis.	**PO:** Bronchospasm: Loading dose: 0.8 mg/kg/dose Maintenance: Birth - 2 months: 3 - 6 mg/kg/day q 8h; 2 - 6 mo: 6 - 15 mg/kg/ day q 6h; 6 - 12 mo: 15 - 22 mg/kg/day q 6h; 1 - 9 yrs: 20 - 22 mg/kg/day q 6h (max. dose 24 mg/kg/day); 12 - 16 yrs: 16 - 18 mg/kg/day q 6h; > 16 yrs: 13 mg/kg/day q 6h (max. dose 900 mg/day) **Dosing is the same for extended release tabs but they are given q 8 - 12h** **PO,IV:** Neonatal apnea: Loading dose: 1 mg/kg for each 2 mcg/ml increase in serum theophylline level desired Maintenance: Preterm infants: 1 mg/kg q 12h; Term infants: 1 - 2 mg/kg q 8h; 4 - 8 weeks postnatal: 1 - 3 mg/kg q 6h **IV:** Bronchospasm: Loading dose: 4.7 mg/kg x 1 dose Maintenance: 6 mo. - 9 yrs: 1.2 mg/kg/hr x 12h then 1 mg/kg/hr; 9 - 16 yrs: 1 mg/kg/hr x 12h then 0.8 mg/kg/hr; > 16 yrs (nonsmoker): 0.7 mg/kg/hr x 12h then 0.5 mg/kg/hr	**CNS:** Headaches, restlessness, dizziness, irritability, insomnia, muscle twitching, <u>seizures</u> **CV:** Palpitations, <u>sinus tachycardia</u>, extrasystoles, flushing, marked <u>hypotension, circulatory failure, cardiac arrest</u> **GI:** Nausea, vomiting, bitter aftertaste, epigastric pain, anorexia, diarrhea **Resp:** Tachypnea **Skin:** Urticaria, exfoliative dermatitis **Other:** Hyperglycemia, SIADH, pain and redness at IV site	**Drugs:** Serum levels decreased by phenytoin and barbiturates; decreases therapeutic effectiveness of lithium and furosemide; may induce bronkospasm when used with beta-adrenergic blockers; decreased hepatic clearance with erythromycin, cimetidine, troleandomycin; increased CNS stimulation with adrenergics; increased metabolism with phenobarbital. **Foods:** Delayed clearance with charcoal-broiled foods.	* Assess respiratory status and vital signs . * Weigh patient. * If child is currently taking theophylline, determine when amount and time last dose given. * Do not allow child to swallow chewable forms whole. * Withhold dose from neonates with heart rate > 180. * Delayed absorption if given with food, but may administer with meals if GI irritation present. * If IV, <u>do not administer faster than 25 mg/minute</u>. * IV administration rate usually 25 - 30 minutes. * Continuous IV rate = 0.9 - 1.5 mg/kg/hr. * Do not use continuous infusion for neonates. * Monitor respiratory status. * Monitor serum drug levels frequently and maintain between 10 - 20 mcg/ml. * Check with pharmacist prior to mixing with any drug. * Incompatible with acid solutions. * Patient/parent education: - Report any CNS, cardiac, or GI side effects to MD. - Monitor respiratory response. - Maintain hydration and weight. - Do not use any OTC drugs containing ephedrine. - Take as directed and at same time each day to maintain levels.

Table 7. CARDIOVASCULAR MEDICATIONS

Name	Uses	Route and Dose	Adverse Reactions/ Side Effects	Drug or Food Interactions	Nursing Considerations
Generic: Atropine **Trade:** Isopto Atropine	Anticholinergic used to treat vagally induced bradycardia, decrease smooth muscle contractions in GI and GU tracts, decrease secretions in respiratory and GI tracts, and occasionally as a bronchodilator.	**PO:** **Antimuscarinic:** 0.01 mg/kg not to exceed 0.4 mg q 4 - 6h **SC:** **Antimuscarinic:** 0.01 mg/kg not to exceed 0.4 mg - may repeat q 4 - 6h **Preop:** < 3kg: 0.1 mg 7 - 9 kg: 0.2 mg 12 - 16 kg: 0.3 mg 20 - 27 kg: 0.4 mg 32 kg: 0.5 mg 41 kg: 0.4 mg **IV:** **Dysrhythmias:** 0.01 - 0.03 mg/kg **Cardiac arrest:** 0.02 mg/kg with a minimum dose of 0.1 mg and maximum dose of 1.0 mg **Inhalation:** 0.05 mg/kg in saline q 6 - 8h	**CNS:** Atropine psychosis, CNS stimulation, restlessness, combativeness, confusion, hallucination, weakness, dizziness, insomnia, headache, paradoxical excitement **CV:** Tachycardia, bradycardia with low doses or slow injection, palpitation **GI:** Nausea, vomiting, loss of taste, bloating, dry mouth, constipation, paralytic ileus **GU:** Urinary retention **Skin:** Hot dry skin, rash, urticaria, dermatitis **Sensory:** Mydriasis, blurred vision, cycloplegia, photophobia, local irritation of eye with topical administration	**Drugs:** Increased effect with MAO inhibitors, increased effects of nitrofurantoin, increased intraocular pressure with other drugs having the same effect, delayed excretion with medications causing urinary alkalinization, decreased absorption with antacids, increased chance of constipation with narcotics. **Foods:** None	• Assess vital signs prior to and frequently following administration. • Give po forms 30 min prior to meals and HS. • Perform good oral hygiene. • Will remain stable for 15 minutes when mixed with other preop medications. • Have patient void before administering preoperatively. • Incompatible with sodium bicarbonate and epinephrine. • Monitor intake and output. • Evaluate bowel sounds and function. • Patient/parent education: - Take only as directed. - Notify MD if side effects occur. - Do not take antacids and antidiarrheals within 1 hour of atropine. - Avoid strenuous activity/exercise. - Avoid hot weather. - Rise to standing position slowly. - Inform of possibility of photophobia. - Avoid operating heavy machinery.

Name	Uses	Route and Dose	Adverse Reactions/ Side Effects	Drug or Food Interactions	Nursing Considerations

Generic: Digoxin
 	
Trade: Lanoxin, Lanoxicaps, S-(-)-digoxin
	Cardiac glycoside used to increase myocardial contractility, increase automaticity, reduce excitability and conduction velocity, and prolong refractory period. Also acts to retain sodium and excrete potassium from myocardium. Used to treat congestive heart failure and to control ventricular rate in atrial flutter and fibrillation.	**PO:**
		Digitalizing Dose:
		Preterm infants: 20 mcg/kg
		Neonates: 30 mcg/kg
		< 2 yrs: 40 - 50 mcg/kg
		2 - 10 yrs: 30 - 40 mcg/kg
		> 10 yrs: 0.75 - 1.25 mg
		These are administered as 1/2 the total dose initially followed by 1/4 the dose q 8 - 18h x 2
		
		Maintenance dose:
		Preterm infants: 5 mcg/kg/day divided q 12h
		Neonates: 8 - 10 mcg/kg/day divided q 12h
		< 2 yrs: 10 - 12 mcg/kg/day divided q 12h
		2 - 10 yrs: 8 - 10 mcg/kg/day divided q 12h
		> 10 yrs: 0.125 - 0.25 mg q day
		
		IV,IM:
		IV or IM doses are 75% of total PO doses except in the > 10 yr group, when IV,IM = PO
			CNS: Tiredness, weakness, headache, confusion, depression, fainting, facial neuralgia, paresthesias, hallucinations, agitation
			CV: Bradycardia, dysrhythmias, hypotension, tachycardia
			GI: Nausea, vomiting, anorexia, stomach pain, diarrhea
			Sensory: Blurred vision, halos
				Drugs: Increased toxicity if used with drugs that cause hypokalemia; increased risk of dysrhythmias if used with other antiarrhythmics, calcium, or sympatho-mimetics; increased levels if used with calcium-channel blocking agents and quinidine; may decrease effects of heparin; increased digoxin needed if on thyroid replacements; reduced absorption with antacids; decreased absorption with chemotherapy and radiation treatments.
				
				Foods: None
					• Assess baseline vital signs and ECG.
					• Obtain baseline serum electrolytes, hepatic and renal function studies.
					• Hydrate if hypovolemic.
					• May take with food.
					• Use calibrated dropper if giving elixir.
					• Ensure that digoxin not digitoxin tablets are administered.
					• Dilute IV doses with at least 4x the volume and administer over at least 5 min.
					• Assess apical pulse for one full minute prior to administering digoxin.
					• Withhold dose if pulse is below normal for age group (often 100 beats/min in children).
					• Monitor ECG during IV administration.
					• Monitor serum electrolytes and hepatic and renal functions, particularly if patient taking diuretics.
					• Monitor serum digoxin levels carefully (levels > 2ng/ml are toxic).
					• Monitor for tachycardia in young children and stomach upset or bradycardia in older children which may indicate toxicity.
					• Patient/parent education:
					  - If ordered by MD, teach parents to assess apical pulse for 1 min prior to administering dose and do so at same time each day.
					  - Notify MD and withhold medication if nausea and vomiting occur.
					  - Teach correct measurement and administration.
					  - Teach signs of congestive heart failure.
					  - Due to high risk of accidental poisoning, keep medication out of reach and have syrup of ipecac available.
					  - Wear medical ID bracelet.

Name	Uses	Route and Dose	Adverse Reactions/ Side Effects	Drug or Food Interactions	Nursing Considerations
Generic: Dobutamine **Trade:** Dobutrex	Catecholamine and cardiac stimulant that increases contractility, stroke volume and cardiac output and decreases peripheral vascular resistance with minimal effects on B/P. Used to treat cardiac failure with resultant low cardiac output.	**IV:** 2.5 - 15 mcg/kg/min	**CNS:** Headache, paresthesia **CV:** Ectopic beats, tachycardia, angina, palpitations, hypertension **GI:** Nausea **Resp:** Dyspnea	**Drugs:** Decreased effects if used with beta-adrenergic blockers; ventricular dysrhythmias with halothane or cyclopropane anesthesia; increased cardiac output and decreased pulmonary wedge pressure with nitroprusside; increased pressor effects if used with MAO inhibitors and tricyclic antidepressants. **Food:** None	• Monitor vital signs including EKG, cardiac output, skin temperature, peripheral pulses and pulmonary wedge pressure at least q 1 hour. • Patient must be continuously monitored and on a cardiac monitor. • Correct hypovolemia prior to starting medication. • Use prepared solutions within 24 hours. • Incompatible with many medications - check with pharmacist prior to mixing with other medications or solutions. • Strict intake and output.
Generic: Dopamine **Trade:** Intropin	Precursor to norepinephrine that increases myocardial contractility, stroke volume, and cardiac output by beta adrenergic action. Will increase renal and coronary arterial perfusion at low doses and will cause vasoconstriction at high doses. Used to treat cardiogenic shock and congestive heart failure.	**IV:** Increased renal and coronary artery perfusion: 1 - 5 mcg/kg/min Increased cardiac output: 5 - 10 mcg/kg/min Increased peripheral vascular resistance and cardiac output: > 10 mcg/kg/min	**CNS:** Nervousness, headache, numbness or tingling of fingers or toes **CV:** Chest pain, hypotension, irregular pulse, hypertension and tachycardia with rapid infusion, bradycardia, palpitations **Resp:** Dyspnea **GI:** Nausea, vomiting **Skin:** Color changes or pain from vasoconstriction, gangrene in extremities with prolonged use, tissue necrosis with necrosis	**Drugs:** Prolonged effects with MAO inhibitors, decreased cardiac effects if used with beta-adrenergics, hypotension and bradycardia with IV phenytoin, increased chance of dysrhythmias with digitalis and guanethidine, ventricular dysrhythmias and hypertension with halothane or cyclopropane anesthetics, potentiates diuretics and thyroid medications. **Foods:** None	• Monitor vital signs including EKG, cardiac output, skin temperature, peripheral pulses and pulmonary wedge pressure at least q 1 hour. • Patient must be continuously monitored and on a cardiac monitor. • Correct hypovolemia prior to starting medication. • Monitor IV frequently for extravasation. • Monitor carefully for decreased circulation in extremities. • Incompatible with alkaline medications - check with pharmacist prior to mixing with other medications or solutions. • Strict intake and output.

Name	Uses	Route and Dose	Adverse Reactions/ Side Effects	Drug or Food Interactions	Nursing Considerations
Generic: Epinephrine **Trade:** Adrenalin Ana-Kit	Natural catecholamine used to induce vasoconstriction, bronchodilation, increased heart rate, and cardiac stimulation. Used in cardiac arrest situations to replace catecholamines for cardiac stimulation.	**IV,Intracardiac:** Cardiac stimulation: 5 - 10 mcg/kg either repeated q 5 min. prn or given continuous IV at a rate of 1 mcg/kg/min. If given continuous IV, may be increased by 0.1 mcg/kg/min but not to exceed 1/5 mcg/kg/minute.	**CNS:** Anxiety, restlessness, dizziness, headache, excitability, weakness,syncope, convulsions, fever, chills **CV:** Tachycardia, palpitations, increased blood pressure, flushing, EKG changes, chest pain, irregular pulse **Resp:** Dyspnea, rebound bronchospasm after withdrawal of inhalation therapy **GI:** Nausea, vomiting **Skin:** Necrosis at injection site with repeated injections; pale cold skin **Sensory:** Blurred vision, enlarged pupils **Other:** Prolonged use can lead to matabolic acidosis	**Drugs:** Additive effects with other sympatho-mimetics; decreased respiratory and cardiac effects with beta adrenergic blockers; severe hypotension and tachycardia if given with rapid-acting vasodilators; decreased effects with antihypertensives; increased cardiac effects observed if given with some general anesthetics; increased cardiac effects with cardiac clygosides, tricyclic antidepressants, antihistamines, and thyroid medications; monitor EKG if given with digitalis; added CNS effects with other CNS stimulants and xanthines; increased insulin needs with diabetes. **Foods:** None	• Baseline vital signs, especially pulse and B/P. • Evaluate and monitor EKG, blood gases, CVP, and urine output. • Use 1 mg/ml solution (1:1000) if giving IV. • Monitor blood glucose in diabetic patients closely.

Name	Uses	Route and Dose	Adverse Reactions/ Side Effects	Drug or Food Interactions	Nursing Considerations
Generic: Isoproterenol **Trade:** Isuprel	Beta-adrenergic stimulant used to reduce peripheral vascular resistance and increase the force of cardiac contractions without vasoconstriction. Will cause bronchodilation and relieve bronchospasm.	**SL (sublingual):** Cardiac stimulant: 5 mg adjusted according to patient response Bronchospasm: 5 - 10 mg TID, not exceeding 30 mg/day **IV:** Dysrhythmia or cardiac arrest: 2.5 mcg/min or 0.1 mcg/kg/min and adjusted according to patient response Status asmaticus: 0.08 - 1.7 mcg/kg/min	**CNS:** Nervousness, weakness, insomnia, dizziness, headache, anxiety **CV:** <u>Palpitations</u>, tachycardia, chest pain, <u>hypotension</u> following a slight rise in B/P, irregular pulse **GI:** Nausea, vomiting, ulcerations, teeth damage from sublingual tablets, dry mouth, parotid edema **Skin:** Pale, cold skin; increased sweating	**Drugs:** Decreased effects with propranolol and other beta - adrenergic blockers; dysrhythmias with general anesthesia; potentiates cardiac effects of epinephrine; possible cardiotoxic effects with theophylline **Foods:** None	• Assess baseline vital signs, ECG, blood gases, CVP, and urine output. • Provide meticulous oral care to avoid mucosal and tooth damage from sublingual administration. • Compatible with most IV solutions. • Most stable in alkaline solutions. • Patient/parent education: - Teach correct administration technique. - Do not exceed recommended dose. - Contact MD if side effects occur. - Perform meticulous oral care. - Notify MD if rebound bronchospasms occur.
Generic: Lidocaine **Trade:** Zylocaine	Antiarrhythmic that depresses myocardial activity and is used to treat ventricular dysrhythmias.	**IV:** Antiarrhythmic: 0.5 - 1.0 mg/kg/bolus repeated prn q 5 - 10 minutes. Maintenance infusion of 10 - 50 mcg/kg/min may be utilized, prn and should not exceed 4 mg/min	**CNS:** Drowsiness, confusion, dizziness, impaired vision, paresthesia, tremors, seizures, <u>coma</u> **CV:** <u>Bradycardia</u>, <u>hypotension</u> **GI:** Nausea, vomiting **Resp:** <u>Respiratory arrest</u> **Sensory:** Tinnitus, visual disturbances **Other:** <u>Hypersensitivity reaction</u>	**Drugs:** Increased cardiac depressant effects with phenytoin, propranolol, other antiarrhythmics; increased hepatic metabolism with phenytoin, decreased effects with barbiturates, increased neuromuscular blocking with succinylcholine; decreased hepatic clearance and toxicity with cimetidine and propranolol. **Foods:** None	• Monitor baseline vital signs. • Have resuscitation equipment readily available. • Do not mix with other medications and solutions. • Monitor for CNS and CV side effects. • Constantly monitor ECG and B/P with IV infusion. • Monitor serum electrolytes. • Monitor serum lidocaine levels.

Table 8. DIURETICS

Name	Uses	Route and Dose	Adverse Reactions/ Side Effects	Drug or Food Interactions	Nursing Considerations
Generic: Chlorothiazide **Trade:** Diuril	Short-acting, potassium sparing diuretic used to treat hypertension and with digitalis to treat congestive heart failure.	**PO:** **< 6 mo:** 10 - 33 mg/kg/day in 1 - 2 doses **> 6 mo:** 10 - 22 mg/kg/day in 1 - 2 doses	**CNS:** Fatigue, headache, weakness, mood changes **CV:** Orthostatic hypotension, irregular pulse **GI:** Nausea, vomiting, anorexia, abdominal cramping, dry mouth, thirst **Hepatic:** Hepatic dysfunction **Metabolic:** Hypokalemia, hyponatremia, hypochloremic alkalosis, hyperuricemia, hypercalcemia, hypophosphatemia, hyperglycemia, glycosuria in diabetic patients **Hemic:** Thrombocytopenia, eosinophilia **Other:** Hypersensitivity reaction	**Drugs:** Increased susceptibility to digitalis toxicity and blocking effects of neuromuscular blocking agents due to hypokalemia; added risk of hypokalemia when administered with other drugs having the same effect; possible hyperglycemia with diabetic patients; added effects with other drugs causing orthostatic hypotension. **Foods:** None	* Assess baseline vital signs, CBC, serum electrolytes and glucose, uric acid, weight prior to administration. * Administer po form in early am and prior to meals. * Monitor hydration status. * Monitor blood glucose carefully in diabetic patients. * Monitor for signs of hypokalemia. * Patient/parent education: - Take early in the day and at the same time each day. - May take with food. - Eat potassium rich foods while taking this drug. - Get up slowly to avert orthostatic hypotension. - Avoid added sodium. - Avoid OTC medications that may contain sodium. - Monitor weight and report changes to MD. - Avoid exposure to sun. - Monitor for nausea, vomiting, and diarrhea and report to MD. - If diabetic, monitor blood glucose carefully.

Name	Uses	Route and Dose	Adverse Reactions/ Side Effects	Drug or Food Interactions	Nursing Considerations
Generic: Furosemide **Trade:** Lasix	Rapid acting loop diuretic that works to inhibit sodium reabsorption at the Loop of Henle. Increases potassium excretion in distal tubules. Used to treat edema that accompanies renal failure, congestive heart failure, cerebral edema, pulmonary edema, congenital heart disease, and nephrotic syndrome.	**PO:** 2 mg/kg, increased by 1 - 2 mg/kg q 6 - 8h prn; should not exceed 6 mg/kg/day **IV:** Diuretic: 1 mg/kg, increased by 1 mg/kg q 2h prn; should not exceed 6 mg/kg/day	**CNS:** Vertigo, tinnitus, headache, confusion, fatigue **CV:** Orthostatic hypotension, irregular or weak pulse **GI:** Nausea, vomiting, dry mouth, thirst, stomach pain, diarrhea, anorexia **Hepatic:** Jaundice, hepatic dysfunction **GU:** Profound diuresis **Metabolic:** Hypokalemia, hyponatremia, hypochloremic alkalosis **Sensory:** Tinnitus, deafness, vision changes, photosensitivity **Hemic:** Thrombocytopenia, neutropenia, anemia, leukopenia, aplastic anemia, agranulocytosis	**Drugs:** Increased risk of ototoxicity if used with other drugs having the same risk; increased diuretic effects with indomethacin; increased risk of digitalis toxicity; potentiated effects with other diuretics; prolongs action of neuromuscular blockading agents; decreased lithium clearance; inhibits anticoagulants. **Foods:** None	• Assess baseline vital signs, hydration status, and serum electrolytes. • Weigh patient. • Give po forms in the am to prevent nocturia and with food to decrease gastric upset. • Do not mix IV preparation with acidic solutions. • Do not give IV faster than 4 mg/min to avoid risk of hearing loss. • Daily weights. • Monitor B/P regularly. • Monitor I&O. • Monitor diabetic patients closely for hyperglycemia. • Patient/parent education: - Take at the same time each day and no later than 3 p.m. to avoid nocturia. - Take with food. - Avoid hot tubs, strenuous exercise, hot weather, and alcohol. - Avoid rapid position changes to avert postural hypotension. - Teach patient to recognize and report signs of electrolyte imbalance. - Notify MD of GI symptoms. - Eat potassium-rich foods.

Name	Uses	Route and Dose	Adverse Reactions/ Side Effects	Drug or Food Interactions	Nursing Considerations
Generic: Mannitol **Trade:** Osmitrol	Osmotic diuretic that works by increasing plasma osmolality, thus increasing water loss from tissues. Also facilitates water loss and toxin excretion from kidneys. Used to reduce edema in acute renal failure, cerebral and pulmonary edema, to decrease intraocular pressure, and to facilitate excretion of toxic substances resulting from overdose.	**IV:** Diuretic: 2 g/kg in 15 - 20% solution over 2 - 6h Cerebral edema, increased ICP, glaucoma: 1 - 2 g/kg in 15 - 20% solution over 30 - 60 min Overdose: up to 2 g/kg in 5 - 10% solution	**CNS:** Confusion, paresthesia, weakness, headache, dizziness, blurred vision, <u>seizures</u> **CV:** Chest pain, <u>tachycardia</u> **Resp:** Dyspnea, wheezing, coughing **GI:** Nausea, vomiting, thirst **GU:** Increased urination, <u>renal failure</u> following large doses urinary retention, edema **Skin:** Rash, hives, edema and/or necrosis with extravasation **Metabolic:** Hypovolemia, hyponatremia, hyperkalemia	**Drugs:** Potentiates other diuretics; hypokalemia may increase risk of digitalis toxicity; increases lithium excretion. **Food:** None	• Monitor baseline vital signs and serum electrolytes. • Weigh patient daily. • Assess hydration status. • Monitor vital signs and serum electrolytes frequently. • I&O. • Monitor for signs of hypovolemia and electrolyte imbalances. • Avoid extravasation. • Monitor for signs of rebound increased intracranial or intraocular pressure, which may occur approximately 12h following cessation of therapy.
Generic: Spironolactone **Trade:** Aldactone	Potassium sparing diuretic, often in combination with chlorothiazide.	**PO:** Hypertension/edema: 3.3 mg/kg/day in 1 - 4 doses; may be adjusted upward prn after 5 days of therapy	**CNS:** Lethargy, confusion, fatigue, dizziness, headache **CV:** <u>Dysrhythmias</u> **GI:** Nausea, vomiting, anorexia, abdominal cramping, diarrhea, dry mouth, thirst **Hepatic:** Elevated BUN **GU:** Menstrual abnormalities, breast enlargement **Metabolic:** <u>Hyperkalemia</u>, <u>metabolic acidosis</u>, hyponatremia **Skin:** Rash, urticaria, sweating	**Drugs:** Hypoglycemia in patients on insulin; hyperkalemia with potassium supplements, captopril; reduced excretion of digoxin; inhibited inotropic effects of digitalis; decreased effects with salicylates; potassium excretion potentiated with corticosteroids; potentiated by other diuretics; reduced clearance of lithium; potentiated by other potassium sparing drugs **Foods:** None	• Assess and monitor baseline vital signs, CBC, BUN, creatinine, ECG, serum electrolytes, and weight. • Tablets may be compounded into a suspension. • Refrigerate suspension and discard after 1 month. • Give with food. • Monitor for signs of hyperkalemia. • Monitor blood glucose in diabetic patients. • Patient/parent education: - Avoid potassium rich foods. - Teach signs of hyperkalemia. - Report any adverse effects to MD.

Table 9. GASTROINTESTIONAL MEDICATIONS

Name	Uses	Route and Dose	Adverse Reactions/ Side Effects	Drug or Food Interactions	Nursing Considerations

Generic: Aluminum Hydroxide
 	
Trade: Mylanta
	Antacid that neutralizes gastric acid. Used to treat gastritis and peptic ulcers.	**PO:**
		Ulcer: 5 - 15 ml/dose q 3 - 6h or 1 - 3h following meals and HS
		Prophylaxis against GI Bleeding: infants: 2 - 5 ml/dose q 1 - 2h children: 5 - 15 ml/dose q 1 - 2h
			GI: Constipation, anorexia, intestinal obstruction, fecal impaction
			Other: Hypophosphatemia, hypercalciuria, dementia resulting from aluminum toxicity
				Drugs: Interferes with absorption of tetracyclines, digoxin, phenytoin, isoniazid, iron, and chlorpromazine.
				
				Foods: None
					• Shake suspension well prior to administering and follow dose with a small amount of water or milk.
					• Chew tablets well to ensure maximum absorption.
					• If given per feeding tube, validate tube placement and patency prior to administering and flush with water following dose.
					• Monitor for constipation.
					• Maintain fluid intake for age.
					• Patient/parent education:
					  - Take only in amount and frequency scheduled.
					  - Monitor for constipation.
					  - Maintain fluid intake.
					  - Avoid OTC drugs with MD permission.

Generic: Cimetidine
 	
Trade: Tagamet
	Antihistamine that reduces acid secretion in the stomach by interfering with HCl receptor sites. Used to treat GI hemor-rhage, peptic ulcer, hyper-secretory syn-drome, GE reflux, and as adjunct with severe pan-creatic insuf-ficiency that fails to respond to oral pancreatic enzyme supplements.	**PO:**
		20 - 40 mg/kg/day q 6h, following meals and HS
		
		IM,IV:
		20 - 40 mg/kg/day q 6h.
		Max dose = 2400 mg/day
			CNS: Dizziness, headache, agitation, restlessness, confusion, depression, delirium, hallucinations
			CV: Bradycardia, hypotension
			GI: Mild, transient diarrhea
			Hepatic: Increase in SGOT, SGPT, alkaline phosphatase
			GU: Transient rise in serum creatinine, BUN
			Hemic: Neutropenia, agranulocytosis, thrombocytopenia, aplastic anemia
			Endocrine: Mild gynecomastia following 1 month of treatment
			Other: Muscular pain
				Drugs: Decreased action if given with antacids; potentiates warfarin; reduces hepatic metabolism of phenytoin, lidocaine, and theophylline; decreased effectiveness with smoking
				
				Foods: None
					• Assess stool quantity and quality with cystic fibrosis patients.
					• Assess PT if on warfarin therapy.
					• Usually given 1 hour prior to meals.
					• Do not give with antacids.
					• Do not administer IM or IV if precipitate or discoloration of preparation noted.
					• IM injection painful.
					• Must dilute prior to IV administration.
					• Infuse over at least 2 minutes.
					• Monitor for side effects.
					• Patient/parent education:
					  - Follow prescribed regime.
					  - Avoid sudden stoppage of drug to avoid ulcer perforation.
					  - Notify MD of side effects.
					  - Continue follow-up with MD.
					  - Do not take OTC drugs with MD permission.

Name	Uses	Route and Dose	Adverse Reactions/ Side Effects	Drug or Food Interactions	Nursing Considerations
Generic: Glycopyrrolate **Trade:** Robinul	Synthetic anticholinergic used to inhibit GI and GU motility and decrease folume of gastric and pancreatic secretions. Used in management of peptic ulcer and other GI diseases associated with hyperacidity, hypermotility, and spasm.	**PO:** > 12 yr: 1 mg TID. Max dose = 8 mg/day **IM, IV:** 0.1 - 0.2 mg as a single dose	**CNS:** Drowsiness, weakness, dizziness **CV:** Palpitation, tachycardia **GI:** Constipation **GU:** Urinary hesitancy or retention **Sensory:** Blurred vision **Other:** Decreased sweating	**Drugs:** Incompatible with chloramphenicol, diazepam, sodium pentobarbital, sodium bicarbonate, or other drugs that may raise pH > 6. **Food:** None	• Monitor vital signs. • Monitor I & O. • Patient/parent education: - Avoid high environmental temperature. - Avoid operating heavy machinery. - Take only as directed. - Report adverse side effects to MD.
Generic: Metoclopromide Hydrochloride **Trade:** Reglan	Antiemetic used to treat GE reflux.	**PO,IV:** **1 - 6 yr:** 0.1 mg/kg/dose q 6h **6 - 14 yr:** 2.5 - 5 mg/dose q 6h **> 14 yr:** 10 mg/dose	**CNS:** Restlessness, lassitude, drowsiness, fatigue, insomnia, dizziness, headache, extrapyramidal symptoms **CV:** Transient hypertension **GI:** Constipation, diarrhea, dry mouth **Skin:** Maculopapular rash, urticaria, glossal or periorbital edema	**Drugs:** Potentiates depressive effects of opiates, analgesics, anticolinergics, sedatives, alcohol, barbiturates, and tranquilizers; decreased absorption of digoxin; increased absorption of acetaminophen, salicylates, diazepam, ethanol, levodopa, lithium, and tetracycline; increased incidence of extrapyramidal side effects with phenothiazines and butyrophenones. **Foods:** None	• Assess and monitor baseline vital signs. • Give 30 minutes prior to meals and HS for GE reflux. • Give slow IV push over at least 2 minutes. • Protect intermittent IV infusion bags from light. • Consult pharmacist prior to mixing with any other drug. • Monitor for extrapyramidal reactions 24 to 48 hours after administration. • Treat extrapyramidal reactions with diaphenhydramine. • Patient/parent education: - Teach side effects. - Teach proper administration.

Name	Uses	Route and Dose	Adverse Reactions/ Side Effects	Drug or Food Interactions	Nursing Considerations
Generic: Ranitidine Hydrochloride **Trade:** Zantac	Antihistamine that prohibits HCl secretion by binding with HCl receptor sites. Used to treat active GI hemorrhage, peptic ulcer disease, hypersecretory syndrome, and GE reflux.	**PO:** 2 - 4 mg/kg/day divided q 12h **IM, IV:** 1 - 2 mg/kg/day divided q 6 - 8h	**CNS:** Headache, dizziness, malaise, insomnia **CV:** Bradycardia, tachycardia **GI:** Nausea, constipation, abdominal discomfort **Hepatic:** Increase in SGOT, SGPT, alkaline phosphatase, LDH, total bilirubin, jaundice **Skin:** Maculopapular rash, urticaria, pruritus **Hemic:** Leukopenia, granulocytopenia, agranulocytosis, thrombocytopenia **Other:** Hypersensitivity reaction	**Drugs:** Decreased action with antacids; decreased absorption and increased serum levels of ranitidine with propantheline bromide; decreased effectiveness with smoking. **Foods:** None	• May give with meals. • If only given once per day, give HS for best results. • Do not use IM or IV preparation if discolored or contains precepitate. • Dilute IV to a concentration of 2 mg/ml and give slowly. • Assess for side effects. • Assess effectiveness. • Patient/parent education: - Follow prescribed dosage and administration times. - Notify MD if side effects occur. - Continue follow-up with MD. - Do not take OTC drugs without MD permission. - Adhere to prescribed diet.

Table 10. STEROIDS

Name	Uses	Route and Dose	Adverse Reactions/ Side Effects	Drug or Food Interactions	Nursing Considerations
Generic: Dexamethasone **Trade:** Decadron	Corticosteroid used for its anti-inflammatory, immunosuppressant, and metabolic effects. Used for collagen, dermatologic, allergic, and leukemic diseases, as replacement therapy in adrenocortical deficiencies, and in inhaler form with asthma and rhinitis.	**PO:** 0.024 - 0.34 mg/kg/day q 6h **IM,IV:** Increased ICP: loading dose = 0.5 - 1.5 mg/kg then 0.2 - 0.5 mg/kg/day q 6h x 5 doses and tapered over 5 days Airway edema: 0.25 - 0.5 mg/kg/day q 6h prn croup or 24h prior to planned extubation followed by 4 - 6 additional doses **Ophthalmic:** Drops: 1 drop q 6 - 8h, up to q 4h Ointment: 1 cm q 6 - 8h **Otic:** 3 - 4 drops (ophthalmic solution) q 8 - 12h **Inhalation:** 2 inhalations q 6 - 8h (max. = 8 inhalations/day) **Topical:** Apply thin film 1 - 4 times/day	**CNS:** Headache, vertigo, euphoria, insomnia, increased ICP, psychotic behavior, seizures **CV:** Edema, hypertension, congestive heart failure **GI:** Nausea, vomiting, change in appetite, GI irritation, abdominal distention, pancreatitis, ulcerative esophagitis, peptic ulcer **Skin:** Impaired wound healing, fragile skin, petechia, ecchymosis, acne, facial erythema, increased sweating, burning, itching, irritation, dryness, folliculitis, hypertrichosis, hypopigmentation, allergic contact dermatitis, maceration, secondary infection, skin atrophy, striae, miliaria **Hemic:** Thrombocytopenia **Endocrine:** HPA-axis suppression, menstrual irregularities, Cushing's states, secondary adrenocortical insufficiency, pituitary unresponsiveness **Musculoskeletal:** Bone growth suppression, osteoporosis, muscle weakness, aseptic necrosis of femoral and humeral heads **Sensory:** Posterior subcapsular cataracts, increased intraocular pressure **Other:** Sodium retention, negative nitrogen balance, hypokalemia, hyperglycemia, increased susceptibility to infections	**Drugs:** Increased risk of hepatotoxicity with high doses of acetaminophen; decreased risk of gastric ulceration with analgesics and antiinflammatory drugs; increased risk of hypokalemia with amphotericin B and potassium-depleting diuretics; decreases effects of anticoagulants; lowered seizure threshold with anticonvulsants; may potentiate live virus vaccines. **Foods:** None	• Obtain baseline weight and height. • Do not use ophthalmic preparation if eye is infected. • Do not use during acute asthma attack. • Take with food to decrease GI irritation. • Do not give IM doses in deltoid muscle. • May give slow IV push. • Incompatible with some IV solutions and drugs - check with pharmacist prior to mixing. • Monitor B/P during IV infusion. • Observe for side effects. • Patient/parent education: - Take medication only as directed. - Do not alter dosage or stop suddenly. - Demonstrate administration of all forms other than po. - Monitor for and report adverse effects. - Check weight daily and report sudden changes to MD. - Have eyes checked q 6 weeks if on long-term therapy. - Do not get skin tests or vaccinations during therapy. - Observe for signs of infection. - Do not use OTC medications. - Do not use inhaler during asthma attack. - Have child carry medical identification card.

Name	Uses	Route and Dose	Adverse Reactions/ Side Effects	Drug or Food Interactions	Nursing Considerations
Generic: Hydrocortisone **Trade:** CaldeCORT, Cortef, Hydrocortone	Short-acting glucocortico-steroid used for its antiinflamma-tory, immunosup-pressant, and metabolic actions. Used to treat collagen, dermatologic, and allergic disorders.	**PO:** 0.56 - 8 mg/kg/day divided q 6 - 8h **IM:** 0.16 - 1 mg/kg/day divided q 12 - 24h **IV:** 0.16 - 1 mg/kg/day divided q 12 - 24h Adrenal Insufficiency: 1 - 2 mg/kg per dose x 1 then 25 - 50 mg/day for infants and 150 - 250 mg/day for children in divided doses. Status asthmaticus: loading of 4 - 8 mg/kg then 8 mg/kg/day divided q 6h **Topical:** Lotion: 0.25%, 0.5%, or 1% solutions - apply sparingly q 12 - 24h; 2.5% apply q day, Cream: 0.1%, 0.25%, 0.5% or 1% solutions - apply thin film q 12 - 24h Ointment: 0.1%, 0.5%, or 1% - apply thin film q 12 - 24h; 0.2% or 2.5% applied q day	**CNS:** Headache, vertigo, euphoria, insomnia, in-creased ICP, psychotic behavior, seizures **CV:** Edema, hypertension, CHF **GI:** Nausea, vomiting, change in appetite, GI irritation, abdominal distension, pancreatitis, ulcerative esophagitis, peptic ulcer **Skin:** Impaired wound heal-ing, thin fragile skin, pete-chiae, ecchymosis, acne, facial redness, increased sweating, folliculitis, hyper-trichosis, hypopigmenta-tion, allergic contact dermatitis, maceration, secondary infection, skin atrophy, striae, miliaria **Endocrine:** HPA-axis suppression, menstrual irregularities, Cushing's states, secondary adreno-cortical or pituitary unresponsiveness **Musculoskeletal:** Suppressed bone growth, osteoporosis, muscle weak-ness, aseptic necrosis of femoral and humeral heads **Other:** Sodium retention, potassium loss, suscep-tibility to infections, hyper-glycemia, hypokalemia, withdrawal	**Drugs:** Increased risk of hepatotoxicity with high doses of acetaminophen; decreased risk of gastric ulceration with analgesics and antiinflammatory drugs; increased risk of hypoka-lemia with amphotericin B and potassium-depleting diuretics; decreases effects of anticoagulants; lowered seizure threshold with anticonvulsants; may potentiate live virus vaccines. **Foods:** None	• Obtain baseline weight and height. • Take with food to decrease GI irrita-tion. • Do not give IM doses in deltoid muscle. • May give slow IV push. • Incompatible with some IV solu-tions and drugs - check with phar-macist • Monitor B/P during IV infusion. • Observe for side effects. • Patient/parent education: - Take medication only as directed. - Do not alter dosage or stop sud-denly. - Demonstrate administration of all forms other than po. - Monitor for and report adverse effects. - Check weight daily and report sud-den changes to MD. - Do not get skin tests or vaccina-tions during therapy. - Observe for signs of infection. - Do not use OTC medications. - Have child carry medical identification card.

Name	Uses	Route and Dose	Adverse Reactions/ Side Effects	Drug or Food Interactions	Nursing Considerations
Generic: Methylpredniso- lone **Trade:** Solu-medrol	Intermediate- acting glucocorticoid with strong antiinflammatory and immunosup- pressant actions. Used to treat diseases of endocrine, integu- mentary, colla- gen, and immune systems.	**PO:** Adrenocortical insufficiency: 0.117 - 1.66 mg/kg/day divided q 6 - 8h Antiinflammatory, immuno- suppression: 0.4 - 1.67 mg/kg/day divided q 6 - 8h **IM:** 0.03 - 0.2 mg/kg q 12 to 24h **IV:** Status asthmaticus: initially 1 - 2 mg/kg/dose followed by 1.6 mg/kg/day q 6h **Rectal:** 0.5 - 1 mg/kg q 1 - 2 days for 2 or more weeks **Topical:** Apply thin film q 12 - 24h	**CNS:** Headache, vertigo, euphoria, insomnia, increased ICP, psychotic behavior, seizures **CV:** Edema, hypertension, CHF **GI:** Nausea, vomiting, change in appetite, GI irritation, abdo- minal distension, pancreatitis, ulcerative esophagitis, peptic ulcer **Skin:** Impaired wound heal- ing, thin fragile skin, petechiae, ecchymosis, acne, facial redness, increased sweating, folliculitis, hypertrichosis, hypopigmentation, allergic contact dermatitis, macera- tion, secondary infection, skin atrophy, striae, miliaria **Endocrine:** HPA-axis sup- pression, menstrual irregu- larities, Cushing's states, secondary adrenocortical pituitary unresponsiveness **Musculoskeletal:** Suppressed bone growth, osteoporosis, muscle weak- ness, aseptic necrosis of femoral and humeral heads **Sensory:** Posterior subcap- sular cataracts, increased intraocular pressure **Other:** Sodium retention, potassium loss, susceptibility to infections, hyperglycemia, hypokalemia, withdrawal	**Drugs:** Increased risk of hepatotoxicity with high doses of acetaminophen; decreased risk of gastric ulceration with analgesics and antiinflammatory drugs; increased risk of hypoka- lemia with amphotericin B and potassium-depleting diuretics; decreases effects of anticoagulants; lowered seizure threshold with anticonvulsants; may potentiate live virus vaccines. **Food:** None	• Obtain baseline weight and height. • Take with food to decrease GI irrita- tion. • Do not give IM doses in deltoid muscle. • Do not mix IM Depo-Medrol with any other medications. • Inject IM doses deep into muscle. • May have burning and pain with IM injection. Prevent leakage into der- mis and SQ tissues to avert atrophy or abscess. • May give slow IV push. • Do not interchange Solu-Medrol and Solu-Cortef. • Incompatible with some IV solutions and drugs - check with pharmacist prior to mixing. • Monitor B/P during IV infusion. • Do not leave occlusive dressing over topical applications for > 16 hrs due to increase in possible side effects. • Observe for side effects. • Patient/parent education: - Take medication only as directed. - Do not alter dosage or stop suddenly. - Demonstrate administration of all forms other than po. - Monitor for and report adverse effects. - Check weight daily and report sud- den changes to MD. - Have eyes checked q 6 weeks if on long term therapy. - Do not get skin tests or vaccinations during therapy. - Observe for signs of infection. - Do not use OTC medications. - Have child carry medical identification card.

Name	Uses	Route and Dose	Adverse Reactions/ Side Effects	Drug or Food Interactions	Nursing Considerations
Generic: Prednisone **Trade:** Delta Cortef, Cortalone	Intermediate-acting glucocorticoid with strong antiinflammatory and immunosuppressant actions. Used to treat diseases of endocrine, integu-mentary, collagen, and immune systems.	**PO:** 0.14 - 2 mg/kg/day divided q 6 h **Nephrosis:** 2 mg/kg/day q 6 - 8 h either for 28 days or until urine is protein free x 5 days. If proteinuria persists, may use 4 mg/kg/day q other day for 28 days. **Maintenance:** 2 mg/kg/dose q other day x 28 days and tapered over 4 - 6 weeks **Asthma:** Acute - 0.5 - 1 mg/kg/day x 3 - 5 days. Severe - 5 - 10 mg/day.	**CNS:** Euphoria, insomnia, psychotic behavior **CV:** Edema, hypertension, CHF **GI:** Nausea, vomiting, change in appetite, GI irritation, pancreatitis, peptic ulcer **Skin:** Impaired wound healing, thin fragile skin, petechiae, ecchymosis, acne, facial redness, increased sweating **Hemic:** Thrombocytopenia **Endocrine:** HPA-axis suppression, menstrual irregularities, Cushing's states, secondary adrenocortical pituitary unresponsiveness **Musculoskeletal:** Suppressed bone growth, osteoporosis, muscle weakness **Sensory:** Posterior subcapsular cataracts, increased intraocular pressure **Other:** Negative nitrogen balance, sodium retention, susceptibility to infections, hyperglycemia, hypoka-lemia, withdrawal	**Drugs:** Increased risk of hepatotoxicity with high doses of acetaminophen; decreased risk of gastric ulceration with analgesics and antiinflammatory drugs; increased risk of hypokalemia with amphotericin B and potassium-depleting diuretics; decreases effects of anticoagulants; lowered seizure threshold with anticonvulsants; may potentiate live virus vaccines. **Foods:** None	• Obtain baseline weight and height. • Obtain ECG, chest and spinal X-rays, glucose tolerance test, and an evaluation of HPA-axis function prior to beginning long term therapy. • Assess response to medication. • Encourage good dental care. • Observe for side effects. • Patient/parent education: - Take medication only as directed. - Do not alter dosage or stop suddenly. - Demonstrate administration of all forms other than po. - Monitor for and report adverse effects. - Check weight daily and report sudden changes to MD. - Have eyes checked q 6 weeks if on long term therapy. - Do not get skin tests or vaccinations during therapy. - Observe for signs of infection. - Do not use OTC medications. - Have child carry medical identification card.

Table 11. OTHER MEDICATIONS

Name	Uses	Route and Dose	Adverse Reactions/ Side Effects	Drug or Food Interactions	Nursing Considerations
Generic: Diphenhydramine **Trade:** Benadryl	Antihistamine that works by blocking histamine release. Will not reverse histamine-related response. Used to treat allergic reactions, motion sickness, vertigo, pruritus, and as a sleeping aid.	**PO:** < 9.1 kg: 6.25 - 12.5 mg q 4 - 6h > 9.1 kg: 12.5 - 25 mg q 4 - 6h **PO,IM,IV:** 5 mg/kg/day divided q 6 - 8h (max. dose = 300 mg/day) **Topical:** > 2 yrs: apply TID - QID **OTC:** **Not recommended for children < 6 yrs** Allergy, motion sickness: 6 - 12 yr: 12.5 - 25 mg q 4 - 6h (max. dose = 300 mg/day) > 12 yr: 25 - 50 mg q 4 - 6h (max. dose = 150 mg/day) Cough suppressant: 6 - 12 yr: 12.5 mg q 4h (max. dose = 75 mg/day) > 12 yr: 25 mg q 4h (max. dose = 150 mg/day) Sleeping aid: > 2 yr: 50 mg 20 min. prior to bed; do not use longer than 2 weeks	**CNS:** Altered consciousness ranging from drowsiness to deep sleep, dizziness, headaches, paradoxical excitement, restlessness, insomnia, tremors, euphoria, delirium, seizures **CV:** Palpitations, hypertension, hypotension, cardiovascular collapse **GI:** Dry mouth, nausea, vomiting, diarrhea, constipation **Resp:** Thickened bronchial secretions, nasal stuffiness, wheezing **GU:** Dysuria, urinary retention **Skin:** Photosensitivity, eczema, pruritus, papular rash, contact dermatitis **Hemic:** Leukopenia, agranulocytosis, thrombocytopenia, hemolytic anemia **Sensory:** Diplopia	**Drugs:** Potentiates depressive effects of opiates, analgesics, anticholinergics, sedatives. alcohol, barbiturates, or tranquilizers; potentiated by MAO inhibitors; potentiates oral anticoagulants. **Foods:** None	• Obtain positive identification of organism prior to starting treatment with this drug. • Obtain baseline BUN, serum creatinine, liver function tests, hematologic tests, and weight. • Do not use reconstituted medication if not clear of precipitate and/or foreign matter. • Do not mix with other medications. • Infuse very slowly (usually over 6 hours). • Protect infusion from light. • Obtain full sets of vital signs (including temperature) q 30 minutes during infusion. • Monitor for cardiovascular collapse. • Assess I & O, weight, potassium, magnesium, BUN, serum creatinine, bilirubin, alkaline phosphatase, and SGOT QD until routine dose established then q week. • Obtain weekly CBC. • Monitor for signs of hypokalemia. • Patient/parent education: - Teach proper application of topical medications. - If no improvement noted in 2 weeks, contact MD. - Treatment may last several months. - May stain clothing. - Remove lotion from hands with soap and warm water. - Remove ointment from hands with cleaning fluid. - Do not apply OTC medications over infected area with consulting MD.

Name	Uses	Route and Dose	Adverse Reactions/ Side Effects	Drug or Food Interactions	Nursing Considerations
Generic: Ipecac Syrup **Trade:** Same	Emetic used to treat accidental poisonings.	**PO:** **6 mo - 1 yr:** 5ml/dose **1 - 5 yr & 25 lbs:** 10 - 15 ml/dose **> 5 -12 yr & 25 lbs:** 15 ml/dose **> 12 yrs:** 30 ml/dose	**CNS:** Lethargy, tremors, seizures, coma **CV:** Tachycardia, dysrhythmias, atrial fibrillation, cardiomyopathy, cardiotoxicity **GI:** Bloody diarrhea, protracted vomiting Side effects are usually related to systemic absorption that occurs when vomiting does not occur. They may also accompany eating disorders which involve using the drug to induce vomiting.	**Drugs:** Activated charcoal will inactivate. **Food:** Delayed onset if given with milk.	• Assess substance ingested, time ingested, amount ingested, and treatment that has occurred. • Assess vital signs. • Notify poison control prior to giving syrup of ipecac. • Do not confuse syrup of ipecac with ipecac fluid-extract! Ipecac fluid-extract has 14 times the potency and may lead to death. • Measure dose carefully. • Give 120 - 240 ml of clear or carbonated fluids with this medication. • Do not give with activated charcoal. • Onset of vomiting is 20 - 30 minutes following administration and will continue for 2 - 3 hours. • Patient/parent education: - If vomiting continues longer than 2 - 3 hours, notify MD. - Syrup of ipecac is nonprescription and widely available. - Keep out of child's reach. - Call poison control prior to inducing vomiting. - Check expiration date prior to administering. - Review accident prevention.

Name	Uses	Route and Dose	Adverse Reactions/ Side Effects	Drug or Food Interactions	Nursing Considerations
Generic: Lindane **Trade:** Kwell, Scabene	Pediculicide used to treat scabies, head lice, body lice, and crab lice.	**Topical:** **Scabies and body lice:** Apply thin layer of 1% from chin down. Be sure to apply under fingernails. Wash off in 6 - 8h. **Head lice:** Shampoo with 15 - 30 ml, leave on 4 - 10 minutes and rinse. May need to reapply in 7 days to remove all newly hatched nits. **Crab lice:** Apply shampoo to pubic areas and leave on 4 minutes before rinsing.	**CNS:** Headache, dizziness, clumsiness, restlessness, irritability, seizures **GI:** Nausea, vomiting, mucosal irritation **Skin:** Local irritation, rash, eczema **Other:** Fatal aplastic anemia, hematologic disorders	**Drugs:** None **Foods:** None	• Wear gloves to apply lindane. • Bathe child prior to treatment. • Apply all over skin including creases, hands, feet, and under fingernails. • Do not apply to face or near urethra. • Bathe child 6 - 8 hours after application. • Check for reinfestation and repeat in 7 days, if necessary. • If shampooing for head lice, use regular shampoo prior to treatment. • It is essential to avoid getting into eyes or mucous membranes. • Leave shampoo on for 4 - 10 minutes. • Rinse hair with a solution of 1/2 water and 1/2 white vinegar or liquid fabric softener and comb through with a fine toothed comb to remove all nits. • May repeat treatment in 7 days. • If eyelashes are infested, treat with petroleum jelly rather than lindane. • Patient/parent education: - All bedding, clothing, and bath linens should be washed in hot water and dried for at least 20 minutes on hot. - Combs and brushes should be soaked in a lindane solution. - All family members should be treated. - Upholstery should be professionally cleaned or cushions may be placed in a sealed plastic bag for 48 hoursthen vacuumed well. - School, day care should be notified. - Recheck the child in 1 week for reinfestation.

Name	Uses	Route and Dose	Adverse Reactions/Side Effects	Drug or Food Interactions	Nursing Considerations
Generic: Insulin **Trade:** Humulin R, Iletin Regular, Regular Iletin I, Regular Pork Insulin **Generic:** Isophane Insulin, Suspension **Trade:** NPH, Beef NPH, Iletin II, Humulin N, Iletin NPH **Generic:** Isophane Insulin, Suspension and Insulin **Trade:** Initard, Mixtard **Generic:** Isophane Insulin, Human, Suspension and Insulin Human **Trade:** Novolin 70/30 **Generic:** Insulin Zinc, Suspension **Trade:** Beef Lente, Iletin II, Humulin L, Lente Iletin I, Lente Insulin **Generic:** Extended Insulin, Zinc Suspension (Ultralente Insulin) Suspension **Trade:** Ultralente, Ultralente Iletin I, Ultralente purified Beef **Generic:** Prompt Insulin Zinc (Semilente) **Trade:** Semilente, Semilente Iletin I, Semilente purified Pork	Endogenous hormone secreted by beta cells in the pancreas that allow glucose transport into the cells.	**Individualized per child. Factors such as stress, illness, activity, and growth periods are considered when adjusting dose(s) to achieve control.	**Skin:** Urticarial reactions resembling allergic reactions; local wheal or indurated area beginning approximately 20 minutes following injection and taking 7 days - 3 months to subside; or insulin lipodystrophy (dimpling and atrophy of fatty tissue) **Endocrine:** Hypoglycemia, somogyi effect (rebound hyperglycemia), hyperglycemia **Other:** Allergic reactions	**Drugs:** Increased blood glucose levels with adrenocorticoids, glucocorticoids, amphetamines, contraceptives, corticotropin, dextrothyroxine, diuretics, epinephrine, glucagon, phenytoin, and thyroid hormone; potentiated hypoglycemic effects with anabolic steroids, androgens, disopyramide, salicylates, antiinflammatory analgesics, alcohol, and beta-adrenergic blocking agents; insulin absorption decreased by smoking. **Foods:** Avoid concentrated sugars, saturated fats, cholesterol, and salt	• Assess for symptoms of hyper- or hypoglycemia. • Assess knowledge level and ability/willingness to manage care. • All brands except concentrated iletin II, U-500 available OTC. • Do not store U-500 with other types of insulin to avoid accidental substitution. • Do not substitute types of insulin or brands of insulin or syringes to avoid inaccurate dosing. • Rotate injection sites. • Record site used in nurses notes. • Allow alcohol to dry on injection site <u>before</u> injecting insulin to avoid precipitation of insulin. • Regular insulin is clear and should not have precipitate. • Regular insulin is the <u>only form</u> that may be given <u>IV</u>. • NPH insulin is cloudy in appearance. • Roll NPH to mix - do not shake to avoid air bubbles. • <u>Always draw up clear (regular) insulin before NPH to avoid contamination of regular insulin.</u> • <u>Do not mix NPH with lente.</u> • Roll lente, ultralente, and semilente to mix - do not shake. • Semilente may only be mixed with lente and ultralente. • Do not use semilente for ketoacidosis. • Monitor child for response (including Somogyi effect). • Monitor fluid balance and serum potassium during diabetic ketoacidosis (DKA). • Ensure that all meals and snacks are given on time. *(con't on next page)*

Name	Uses	Route and Dose	Adverse Reactions/ Side Effects	Drug or Food Interactions	Nursing Considerations
					* Patient/parent education: - Assign one nurse to do education. - Approach teaching/education on correct developmental level for both child and parents. - Involve child in care. - Teach child first, if possible, and have child teach parents. - There should always be extra syringes and a spare vial of insulin for emergencies. - Signs and symptoms of hypo or hyperglycemia. - Meal planning and preparation. - Foot care. - Dental care. - Eye examinations. - Child should wear medical alert jewelry. - School, day care, etc. should be notified and know proper response for hyper and hypoglycemia. - Stress importance of continuing medical follow up.

References

American Hospital Formulary Service. (1992). <u>AHFS drug information '92</u>. (34th ed.). Bethesda, MD: American Society of Hospital Pharmacists.

Bindler, R.M. and Howry, L.B. (1991). <u>Pediatric drugs and nursing implications</u>. Norwalk, CT: Appleton & Lange.

Ford, D.C., Leist, E.R., and Phelps, S.J. (1988). <u>Guidelines for administration of intravenous medications to pediatric patients</u>. (3rd ed.). Bethesda, MD: American Society of Hospital Pharmacists.

Greene, M.G. (Ed.). (1991). <u>The Harriet Lane handbook</u>. (12th ed.). Chicago: Year Book Medical Book Publishers.

Shannon, M.T. and Wilson, B.A. (1992). <u>Drugs and nursing implications</u>. (7th ed.). Norwalk, CT: Appleton & Lange.

Trissel, L.A. (1988). <u>Pocket guide to injectable drugs</u>. Bethesda, MD: American Society of Hospital Pharmacists.

Young, T.E. and Mangum, O.B. (1990). <u>Neofax</u>. (3rd ed.). Columbus, OH: Ross Laboratories.

APPENDIX H

Resource Information

AIDS Hotline 1-800-447-AIDS

American Academy of Pediatrics
Publication Department
P.O. Box 927
141 Northwest Point Rd.
Elk Grove Village, IL 60007

American Burn Association
New York-Cornell Medical Center
525 E. 68th Street, Rm. F758
New York, NY 10021

American Cancer Society
1599 Clifton Road, N.E.
Atlanta, GA 30329

American Celiac Society
58 Musano Court
West Orange, NJ 07502

American Cleft Palate Education Foundation, Inc.
331 Salk Hall
University of Pittsburgh
Pittsburgh, PA 15261

American Diabetes Association, Inc.
2 Park Ave
New York , NY 10010

American Epilepsy Foundation
77 Reservoir Road
Quincy, MA 02169

American Heart Association
205 E. 42nd Street
New York, NY 10017

American Lung Association
1740 Broadway
New York, NY 10019

Arthritis Information Clearinghouse
1314 Spring Street N.W.
Arlington, VA 22209

Association for Children and Adults with Learning Disabilities
4156 Library Road
Pittsburgh, PA 15234

Association for Children with Learning Disabilities
5225 Grace Street
Pittsburgh, PA 15236

Association of Birth Defects in Children
3526 Emerywood Lane
Orlando, FL 32812

Asthma and Allergy Foundation of America
1302 18th Street NW, Ste. 303
Washington, D.C. 20032

Cancer Information Clearinghouse
National Cancer institute
Office of Cancer Communication
Building 31, Room 10-A-18
9000 Rockville, MD 20892

Candlelighters Childhood Cancer Foundation
1312 18th Street N.W., #200
Washington, DC 20036

Cystic Fibrosis Foundation
6931 Arlington Road, #200
Bethesda, MD 20814

Epilepsy Foundation of America
4351 Garden City Dr.
Landrover, MD 20785

Federation for Children with Special Needs, Inc.
120 Boylston Street, Ste. 338
Boston, MA 02116

Immunization Practices Advisory Committee
U.S. Public Health Service
Centers for Diasease Control
Atlanta, GA 30333

Juvenile Diabetes Foundation International
23 E. 26th Street
New York, NY 10010

Leukemia Society of America
733 3rd Avenue
New York, NY 10017

March of Dimes Birth Defects Foundation
1275 Mamaroneck Ave
White Plains, NY 10605

Medic Alert Foundation
P. O. Box 1009
Turlock, CA 95380

Muscular Dystrophy Association, Inc.
810 7th Avenue
New York, NY 10019

National Amputation Foundation, Inc.
1245 150th Street
Whitestone, NY 11357

National Association for Parents of the Visually Impaired, Inc.
P. O. Box 180806
Austin, TX 78718

National Association for Downs Syndrome
P.O. Box 4542
Oak Brook, IL 60522-4542

National Association for Sickle Cell Disease, Inc.
4221 Whilshire Blvd.
Los Angeles, CA 90010

National Association of Patients on Hemodialysis and Transplantation
150 Nassau Street
New York, NY 10038

National Center for Health Statistics
Dept. of Health and Human Services
Public Health Services
3700 East-West Highway
Hyattsville, MD 20782

National Child Safety Council
4065 Page Ave
P. O. Box 280
Jackson, MO 49203

National Diabetes Information Clearinghouse
Box NDIC
Bethesda, MD 20892

National Head Injury Foundation
333 Turnpike Road
Southborough, MA 01772

National Hearing Aid Society
20361 Midlebelt Rd.
Livonia, MI 48152

National Hemophilia Foundation
110 Green Street, Room 406
New York, NY 10012

National Kidney Foundation
116 East 27th Street
New York, NY 10016

National Reye's Syndrome Foundation
P. O. Box RS
Bezonia, MI 49616

National Scoliosis Foundation
P. O. Box 547
Belmont, MA 02178

National Easter Seals Society
70 East Lake Street
Chicago, IL 60601

Parent's Anonymous
7120 Franklin Ave.
Los Angeles, CA 90046

Spina Bifida Association of America
1700 Rockville Pike, Suite 250
Rockville, MD 20852

Sudden Infant Death Syndrome Clearinghouse
1555 Wilson Blvd., Ste 600
Rosslyn, VA 22209

The Compassionate Friends
P. O. Box 3696
Oak Brook, Il 60522-3696

United Cerebral Palsy Association
7 Penn Plaza, Suite 804
New York, NY 10001

United Ostomy Association
36 Executive Park, Suite 120
Irvine, CA 92714

APPENDIX I
Abbreviations Related to Pediatrics

ADD - Attention deficit disorder
ADHD - Attention deficit hyperactivity disorder
ADL - Activity of daily living
AGN - Acute glomerulonephritis
AIDS - Acquired immunodeficiency syndrome
ALL - Acute Lymphocytic leukemia
AML - Acute myelocytic leukemia
ANLL - Acute nonlymphocytic leukemia
ARF - Acute renal failure
ASD - Atrial septal defect
BMT - Bone marrow transplant
BPD - Bronchopulmonary dysplasia
CF - Cystic fibrosis
CHD - Congenital heart defect
CHF - Congestive heart failure
CNS - Central nervous system
COA - Coarctation of the aorta
CP - Cerebral palsy or cleft palate
CPT - Chest physiotherapy
CRF - Chronic
CSF - Cerebrospinal fluid
CVA - Cerebrovascular accident
DDST - Denver developmental screening tool
DPT - Diphtheria, pertussis, tetanus
ECMO - Extracorporeal membrane oxygenation
EMG - Electromyelogram
ESR - Erythrocyte sedimentation rate
FAS - Fetal alcohol syndrome
FB - Foreign body
FTT - Failure to thrive
GER - Gastroesophageal reflux
HIB - Hemophilus influenza, type B
HIV - Human immunodeficiency virus
HTLV-3 - Human T-cell lymphotrophic virus, type 3
IICP - Increased Intracranial pressure
IDDM - Insulin dependent diabetes mellitus, Type I

ITP - Idiopathic thrombocytopenic purpura
JRA - Juvenile rheumatoid arthritis
LTB - Laryngotracheobronchitis
MD - Muscular dystrophy
MI - Mitral insufficiency, myocardial infarction
MMR - Measles, mumps, rubella
MR - Mental retardation
MVA - Motor vehicle accident
NO'FTT - Nonorganic failure to thrive
NHL - Non-Hodgkin's lymphoma
OI - Osteogenesis imperfecta
PDA - Patent ductus arteriosus
PS - Pulmonary stenosis
RDS - Respiratory distress syndrome
RF - Rheumatic fever, renal failure
RSV - Respiratory syncytial virus
TEF - Tracheoesophageal fistula
TGV - Transposition of the great vessels
TOF - Tetralogy of Fallot
TOPV - Trivalent oral polio vaccine
UTI - Urinary tract infection
VCUG - Voiding cystourethrogram
VSD - Ventricular septal defect
VUR - Vesicoureteral reflux

APPENDIX J

The 1992-93 List of NANDA Nursing Diagnoses

Activity Intolerance

Activity Intolerance, High Risk for

Adjustment, Impaired

Airway Clearance, Ineffective

Anxiety

Aspiration, High Risk for

Body Image Disturbance

Body Temperature, High Risk for Altered

Breastfeeding, Effective

Breastfeeding, Ineffective

Breastfeeding, Interrupted

Breathing Pattern, Ineffective

Cardiac Output, Decreased

Caregiver Role Strain

Caregiver Role Strain, High Risk for

Communication, Impaired Verbal

Constipation

Constipation, Colonic

Constipation, Perceived

Coping, Defensive

Coping, Ineffective Individual

Decisional Conflict (Specify)

Denial, Ineffective

Diarrhea

Disuse Syndrome, High Risk for

Diversional Activity Deficit

Dysfunctional Ventilatory Weaning Response

Dysreflexia

Family Coping, Compromised, Ineffective

Family Coping, Disabling, Ineffective

Family Coping, Potential for Growth

Family Processes, Altered

Fatigue

Fear

Fluid Volume Deficit

Fluid Volume Deficit, High Risk for

Fluid Volume Excess

Gas Exchange, Impaired

Grieving, Anticipatory

Grieving, Dysfunctional

Growth and Development, Altered

Health Maintenance, Altered

Health-Seeking Behaviors (Specify)

Home Maintenance Management, Impaired

Hopelessness

Hyperthermia

Hypothermia

Incontinence, Bowel

Incontinence, Functional

Incontinence, Reflex

Incontinence, Stress

Incontinence, Total

Incontinence, Urge

Infant Feeding Pattern, Ineffective

Infection, High Risk for

Injury, High Risk for

Knowledge Deficit (Specify)

Management of Therapeutic Regime (Individual), Ineffective

Noncompliance (Specify)

Nutrition: Less than Body Requirements, Altered

Nutrition: More than Body Requirements, Altered

Nutrition: Potential for More than Body Requirements, Altered

Oral Mucous Membrane, Altered

Pain

Pain, Chronic

Parental Role Conflict

Parenting, Altered

Parenting, High Risk for Altered

Peripheral Neurovascular Dysfunction, High Risk for

Personal Identity Disturbance

Physical Mobility, Impaired

Poisoning, High Risk for

Post-Trauma Response

Powerlessness

Protection, Altered

Rape-Trauma Syndrome

Rape-Trauma Syndrome: Compound Reaction

Rape Trauma Syndrome: Silent Reaction

Relocation Stress Syndrome

Role Performance, Altered

Self-Care Deficit:

  Bathing/Hygiene

  Dressing/Grooming

    Feeding

    Toileting

Self-Esteem, Chronic Low

Self-Esteem, Situational Low

Self-Esteem Disturbance

Self Mutilation, High Risk for

Sensory/Perceptual Alterations (Specify: Visual, Auditory, Kinesthetic, Gustatory, Tactile, Olfactory)

Sexual Dysfunction

Sexual Patterns, Altered

Skin Integrity, Impaired

Skin Integrity, High Risk for

Sleep Pattern Disturbance

Social Interaction, Impaired

Social Isolation

Spiritual Distress (Distress of the Human Spirit)

Suffocation, High Risk for

Swallowing, Impaired

Thermoregulation, Ineffective

Thought Processes, Altered

Tissue Integrity, Impaired

Tissue Perfusion, Altered (Specify Type) (Renal, cerebral, cardiopulmonary, gastrointestinal, peripheral)

Trauma, High Risk for

Unilateral Neglect

Urinary Elimination, Altered

Urinary Retention

Ventilation, Inability to Sustain Spontaneous

Violence, High Risk for: Self-Directed or Directed at Others

APPENDIX K
References

Canobbio, M. (1990). <u>Cardiovascular Disorders</u>. St. Louis: The CV Mosby Company.

Dixon, S. and Stein, M. (1987). <u>Encounters with children -- pediatric behavior and development</u>. Chicago: Year Book Medical Publishers.

Graef, J.W. (Ed.). (1993) <u>Manual of Pediatric Therapeutics</u> (5th ed.). Boston: Little, Brown and Company.

Lanzkowsky, P. (1989). <u>Manual of Pediatric Hematology and Oncology</u>. New York: Churchill Livingstone.

Merenstein, G. and Gardner, S. (1989). <u>Handbook of Neonatal Intensive Care</u> (2nd ed.). St. Louis: The C.V. Mosby Company.

Moore, K. (1977). <u>The developing human: clinically oriented embryology</u>. (2nd ed.). Philadelphia: W.B. Saunders Co.

Mott, S.R., James, S.R., and Sperhac, A.M. (1990). <u>Nursing care of children and families</u>. (2nd ed.). Redwood City, CA: Addison-Wesley.

Rosenstein, B.J., and Fosarelli, P. (1989). <u>Pediatric Pearls: The Handbook of Practical Pediatrics</u>. Chicago: Year Book Medical Publishers, Inc.

Stanhope, M. and Knollmueller, R. (1992). <u>Handbook of Community and Home Health Nursing: Tools for Assessment, Intervention, and Education</u>. St. Louis: Mosby-Year Book.

Whaley, L.F. and Wong, D.L. (1991). <u>Nursing Care of Infants and Children</u> (4th ed.) St. Louis: Mosby-Year Book.

INDEX

A

B

C

I

J

K

L

M

McBurney's point, 54
Measles, 102
Medication administration, 9, 10, 11
Mesoderm, 5
Mononucleosis, 103
Morphine, 4
Mumps, 104
Muscles, 10
Musculoskeletal disorders, 83
Myelomeningocele, 120

N

Naturally acquired active immunity, 99
Naturally acquired passive immunity, 99
Neural tube defect, 120
Neuroblastoma, 143
Nephrotic syndrome, 70
Neurovascular status, 84
Non-Hodgkin's lymphoma, 144

O

Oliguria, 68
Omphalocele, 51
Oncology disorders, 135
Orchioplexy, 67
Osteogenesis, imperfecta, 88
Osteogenic sarcoma, 144
Osteomyelitis, 92
Otitis media, 48, 49

P

Pain, 15, 50
Pancrease, 20
Pancreatic enzymes, 21
Patent ductus arteriosus, 29

Pediculosis capitis, 101
Peritonitis, 54, 55, 59, 61
Pertussis, 100
Phenylketonuria, (PKU), 80
Piaget, 2
Pilocarpine, 20
Pinworms, 101
Plasma, 149
Play, 4
Play therapy, 16
Pneumonia, 30
Poliomyelitis, 104
Preschoolers, 12, 13, 15
Projectile vomiting, 52
Protein, 21
Proximodistal, 2
Pulmozyme, 20
Pulse, 36
Pulse pressure, 36
Pulmonary stenosis, 37
Pyloric stenosis, 52

R

Radiotherapy, 137
Renal system, 65
Respiratory disorders, 19
Respiratory distress syndrome, 29
Restraints, 16
Retinoblastoma, 146
Reye's syndrome, 124
Rhabdomyosarcoma, 146
Rheumatic fever, 43
Ringworm, 155
Roseola, 102
Rubella, 104
Rubeola, 103

Order Form: 1(800) 825-3150
Call, fax or mail to Skidmore-Roth Publishing, Inc.

Qty.	Title	Price	Total
	1994 Nurse's Trivia Calendar	$9.95	
	RN NCLEX Review Cards, 2nd Ed.	$24.95	
	PN/VN Review Cards	$24.95	
	Nurse's Survival Guide, 2nd Ed.	$24.95	
	The Body in Brief, 2nd Ed.	$26.95	
	The OSHA Handbook	$79.95	
	The OBRA Guidelines for Quality Improvement in Long Term Care	$59.95	
	Diagnostic & Laboratory Cards, 2nd Ed.	$23.95	
	Drug Comparison Handbook	$29.95	

Tax of 8.25% applies to Texas residents only. UPS ground shipping $5 for first item, $1 each additional item.		
	Subtotal	
	8.25% Tax	
	Shipping	
	TOTAL	

Name	
Company	
Address	
City	
State	Zip
Phone	

_____ Check enclosed   _____ Visa   _____ MasterCard

Credit Card Number

Card Holder Name

Expiration Date